free yourself from Back Pain

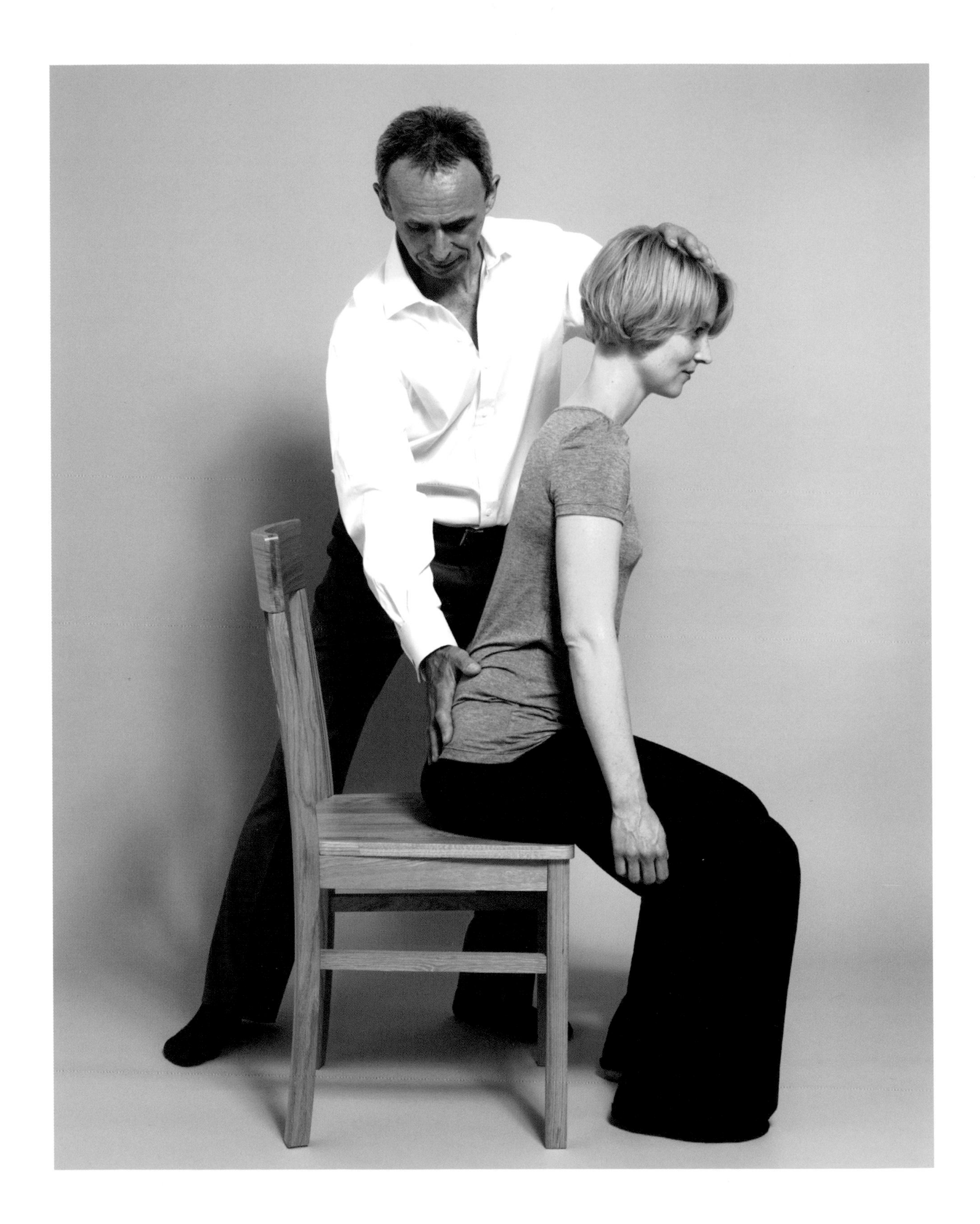

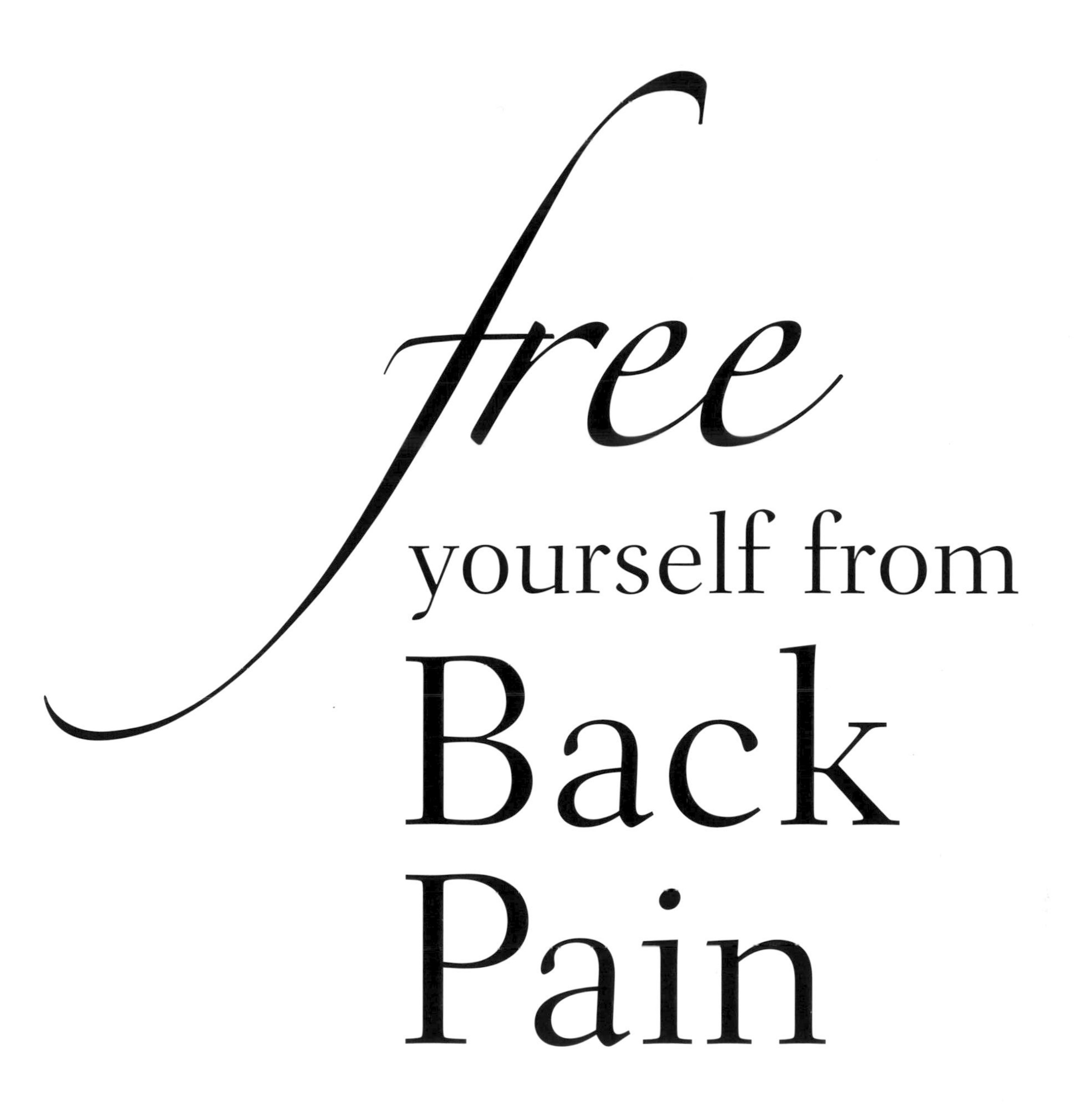

free yourself from Back Pain

a guide to the Alexander Technique

by Noël Kingsley

photography by Eddie Jacob

Kyle Cathie Limited

To Miranda

First published in Great Britain in 2011 by
Kyle Cathie Limited
23 Howland Street,
London W1T 4AY
general.enquiries@kyle-cathie.com
www.kylecathie.com

ISBN 978-1-85626-956-8

Editor: Catharine Robertson
Designer: Louise Leffler
Photographer: Eddie Jacob
Illustrations: Amanda Williams (except p.118 by Philip Wilson)
Copy editor: Barbara Archer
Proofreader: Morag Lyall
Index: Helen Snaith
Production: Gemma John
Models: Elisabeth Dahl, David López Veneros, Susanna Scouller, Angus Antley, Peter French, Gemma John, Jones Antley and Marlie Rowley

A Cataloguing In Publication record for this title is available from the British Library.

Printed and bound in China by C&C Offset Printing Co. Ltd.

Contents

Introduction

Wouldn't relief from back pain be bliss? Even when the pain is short-lived, our period of discomfort can seem like an eternity as the effects of it interfere with almost everything we do, restricting our mobility as we guard against every movement. It can even be isolating, distancing us from our friends and colleagues as we try to cope with the persistent ache or pain. The guidelines and principles of the Alexander Technique presented in this book can change all that and help make your back pain a thing of the past.

It is extraordinary to think that 80 per cent of all adults will experience back pain at some point in their life, and half of the population report low back pain lasting for at least 24 hours at some time in the year.[1] Over 60 million working days are lost each year to absenteeism due to back pain.

Back pain would seem to be something we can expect in today's fast-paced lifestyle and with the hours of deskwork we routinely undertake. In some ways it may be reassuring to know there are a great many others who suffer similarly, but having such awareness cannot make us happy nor does it do anything to alleviate our physical discomfort or change our life for the better.

If you experience back pain it is important to first visit your doctor so that the cause can be diagnosed and suitable treatment prescribed. This may require a trip to the hospital for X-rays, MRI or CT scans to check that there are no serious causes such as over-stressed kidneys or a tumour. However, it is very common for the resulting images to show nothing other than compression or increased curvature of the spine, a disc protrusion or prolapsed disc. We may remember spraining a muscle when reaching up into a bedroom cupboard or bending to pick up groceries in the supermarket; in such instances we probably knew the source of our discomfort. But very often there can be muscle strain of unknown origin which we simply accept. Physiotherapy and a course of prescribed exercises may help. However it is quite possible for us to experience a lingering sensation of weakness, stiffness or mild pain that seems to overshadow our daily life. Although it's possible to keep extreme discomfort at bay, we may never feel that the problem has entirely gone away.

Given the very high number of people who experience back pain, we may be forgiven for thinking this is normal. However it is usually something that we did not suffer from as children, but developed as we got older. Back pain is not a problem in itself, except for the discomfort and the debilitating effect it has on our quality of life, limiting our activities and lowering our performance. Pain of any sort is a warning, it is the body's way of telling us that there is something wrong. Back pain too is an indication that our body is not in the best condition. Most cases of back pain relate to our posture – how we sit, stand, walk, bend and move around in daily life, activities that require us to use all of our hundreds of muscles in a well co-ordinated way. Poor postural habits such as slouching, hunching or stiffening interfere with the subtle and sophisticated working of our muscles, creating unnecessary strain. If such postural habits are the cause of our muscle strain and discomfort, surgical intervention and drugs can be avoided if we can learn to apply the Alexander Technique in our daily lives.

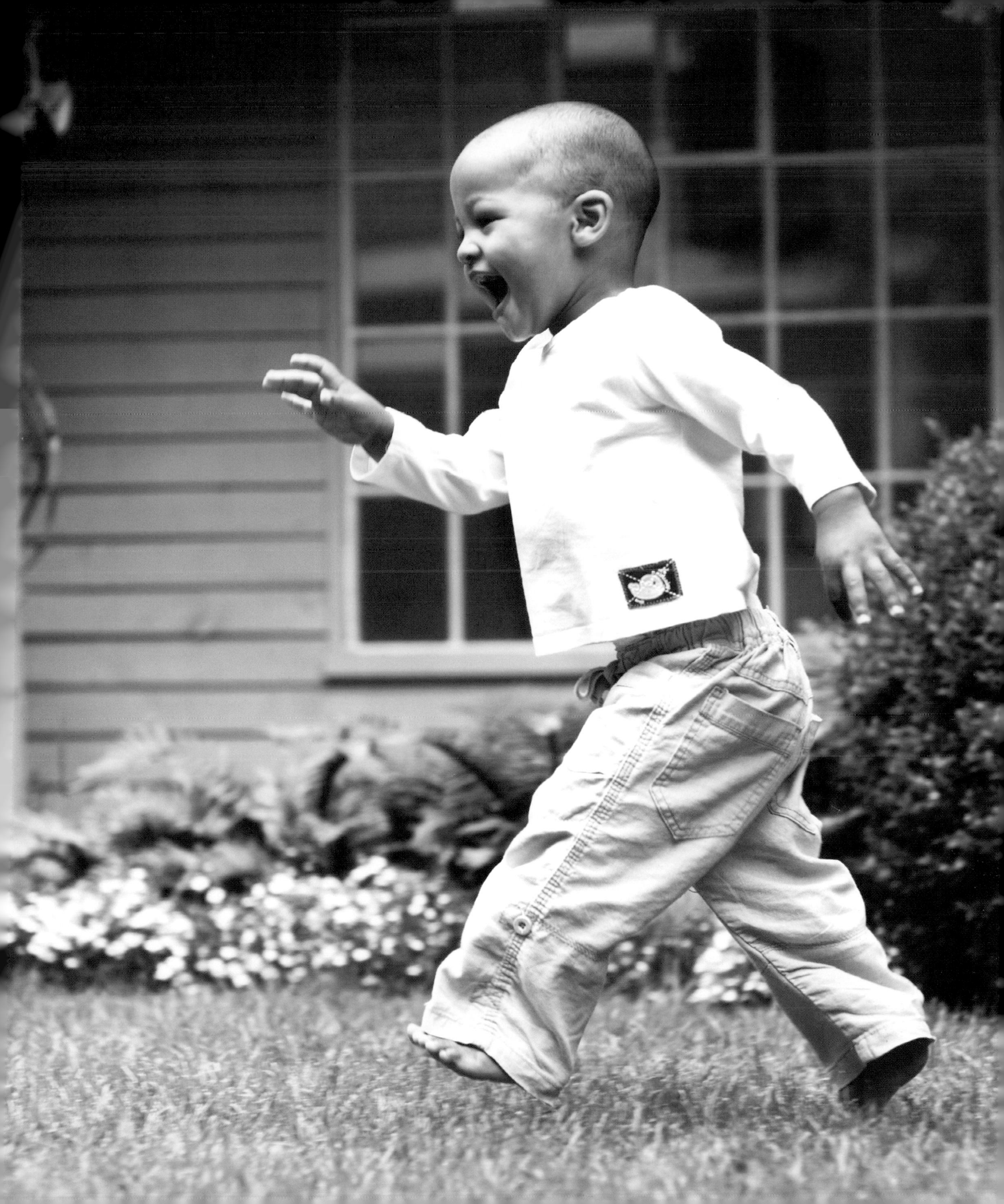

The Alexander Technique

In 2008 a major study by the *British Medical Journal* (*BMJ*) proved that one-to-one lessons in the Alexander Technique from registered teachers provides significant long-term benefits for 'pupils' with chronic low back pain.

The Alexander Technique is a self-help method that enables us to bring about the best 'use' of ourselves in everyday situations. It helps us to observe and inhibit harmful patterns of movement and posture that interfere with the efficient and healthy working of our body. Where instruction in most fields teaches us what to do, the Alexander Technique is about learning what not to do and how to prevent it. It is re-educational and helps us eliminate harmful postural habits, avoid unnecessary strain and enables us to make the most of ourselves: physically and mentally. While the *BMJ* trial showed how successful the Alexander Technique can be in helping overcome the causes of back pain, this is only one of the many benefits. Each and every one of us has a potential for health, well-being and performance way beyond our imagination, and the Alexander Technique offers a means of transformation for almost anyone in any situation.

The Alexander Technique is renowned for helping overcome postural problems, relieving stress, eliminating back pain, neck pain, tension headaches, general stiffness, breathing difficulties, sciatica and many other ailments. Learning the technique can also help overcome shyness and timidity and promote natural confidence, increased height and stature, a better speaking voice and greater agility and stamina. Its positive effect on general health is widespread, so not only do we enjoy a glowing sense of well-being but it can help us to excel in sport, work situations, public speaking, music and even socially. Elimination of postural habits and refinements in our balance and co-ordination can entirely change the way we function. It has even been known to increase earning potential by developing a greater and more confident stature and the ability to cope in stressful business situations.

From a health perspective, the Alexander Technique is not a therapy, as it is not something that you can have treatment in, rather it is an acquired personal skill provided in the form of lessons. It is a unique form of health education that is taught as a self-help method and can bring real improvement to our quality of life.

In order to learn the Alexander Technique so we can apply it ourselves, it is necessary to have a short course of hands-on lessons from a suitably qualified Alexander Technique teacher. As pupils (not patients), we become more aware of our postural habits and learn to release unnecessary tensions, while also allowing ourselves to attain our full height and stature, without any perceived effort. In doing so, we regain much of the natural poise we had as young children. The hands-on guidance in walking, standing, sitting and bending that we receive during the lesson can quickly help us to 'unlearn' bad postural habits. Most of us have little awareness of the habits that are the cause of our discomfort; this becomes very apparent during a lesson when we stop and observe what it is that we are doing that interferes with good 'use'. Rather than learning how to stand, sit and walk, we learn a new 'means-whereby' we can prevent wrong habitual use from interfering, so natural and healthy poise can re-emerge. 'Prevent the wrong thing and the right thing will do itself,' said F.M. Alexander. We begin releasing tension we did not even know existed; we may experience a new way of standing as feeling quite alien and even wrong although strangely comfortable. Hence hands-on one-to-one guidance is usually necessary for progress to be made.

As the nature of Alexander Technique lessons is experiential and mostly involves guided movement, there is no 'note-taking' as such, nor are there many hand-outs or instructions. It is, therefore, the purpose of this book to act as an aide-mémoire, providing helpful advice, tips and further information to accompany the actual lessons. Confidence can be gained from the positive results of the *BMJ* Back Pain Trial which concluded that real relief can be gained from back pain and avoided in the future if we can re-learn how to move without strain. This book will demonstrate how to do just that.

Our body works as a 'whole', involving both mind and body. With the Alexander Technique we learn to become more consciously in control of our whole self, from moment to moment. It helps us be more aware of how we are 'using' ourselves and to be much more present.

While many treatments focus on the region of pain, the Alexander approach is quite different in that it is less direct, but can be much more effective in addressing the fundamental causes of poor posture and pain in a straight-forward and practical manner, helping to restore the free upright poise we enjoyed as young children.

It is our intention with the technique to unlearn postural habits and harmful patterns that upset our co-ordination, which means we are also working on our balance and how we move in relation to gravity. When back pain is caused by poor postural habits (which is by far the most common cause) it is rarely the result of tension limited to the area of pain; this is just the tip of the iceberg. A great many muscles are compensating from moment to moment and if one area is out of natural alignment and balance then other areas of the body will be struggling to adapt. We need to re-train our muscles back into healthy co-ordination.

Whatever reason we may have for enquiring about the Alexander Technique – be it for back pain, other problems or personal performance – the same technique is learnt involving the use of our whole body and mind. We will learn how to maintain healthy upright poise and move in good balance with minimal effort. We have a natural ability to help ourselves by our conscious awareness and potential for controlling how we 'use' our body, to 'inhibit' and prevent harmful tensions and habits. F.M. Alexander referred to this as 'man's supreme inheritance'.[2] The underlying cause of our problems stems from how the many muscles in our body are co-ordinated and this is what we will be addressing with the Alexander Technique. Alexander's method gives us a means of eliminating harmful patterns of movement, while also improving our muscular co-ordination, so the over-stressed muscles do less and underactive muscles do their fair share of work. As our co-ordination improves, our poise will change, our backache will likely disappear and we will move more freely with upright and expansive stature. So, no matter what reason we have for learning the Alexander Technique, by addressing the co-ordination of our muscles and our balance, the results we want – i.e. a pain-free back – will follow.

The Alexander Technique gives us a means of working *indirectly* on our problems; we learn a new 'means-whereby'. It is how we are 'using' ourselves while we sit, stand, walk or bend that causes our problems. Alexander's technique is simple and practical, if a little unusual, but we soon become accustomed to applying the principles of Inhibition and Direction that make profound changes to how we feel and function.

There are no parts of the technique that apply to one person's situation and not another's. The technique in its whole form should be used by everyone, no matter what their particular interest. If you are new to the Alexander Technique and have not had one-to-one lessons from a qualified teacher, you should follow the chapters and guidelines in the sequence given and not skip chapters or omit sections that may seem irrelevant – it's all important. It is hoped that once you are familiar with the technique you will find it helpful to dip into different chapters for guidance.

The exercises in this book allow you to experiment with new ways of thinking and moving, however they are not exercises in the traditional sense of the word as they are not intended to strengthen but to improve co-ordination. Each is an opportunity to develop your awareness and ability using the dual processes we refer to as Inhibition and Direction. They are a 'means-whereby' you can improve your 'use' and functioning by conscious control. Each of these procedures is not an 'end' in itself, but an indirect 'means to an end' and it will help if you adopt an attitude of experimentation and observation of yourself in movement.

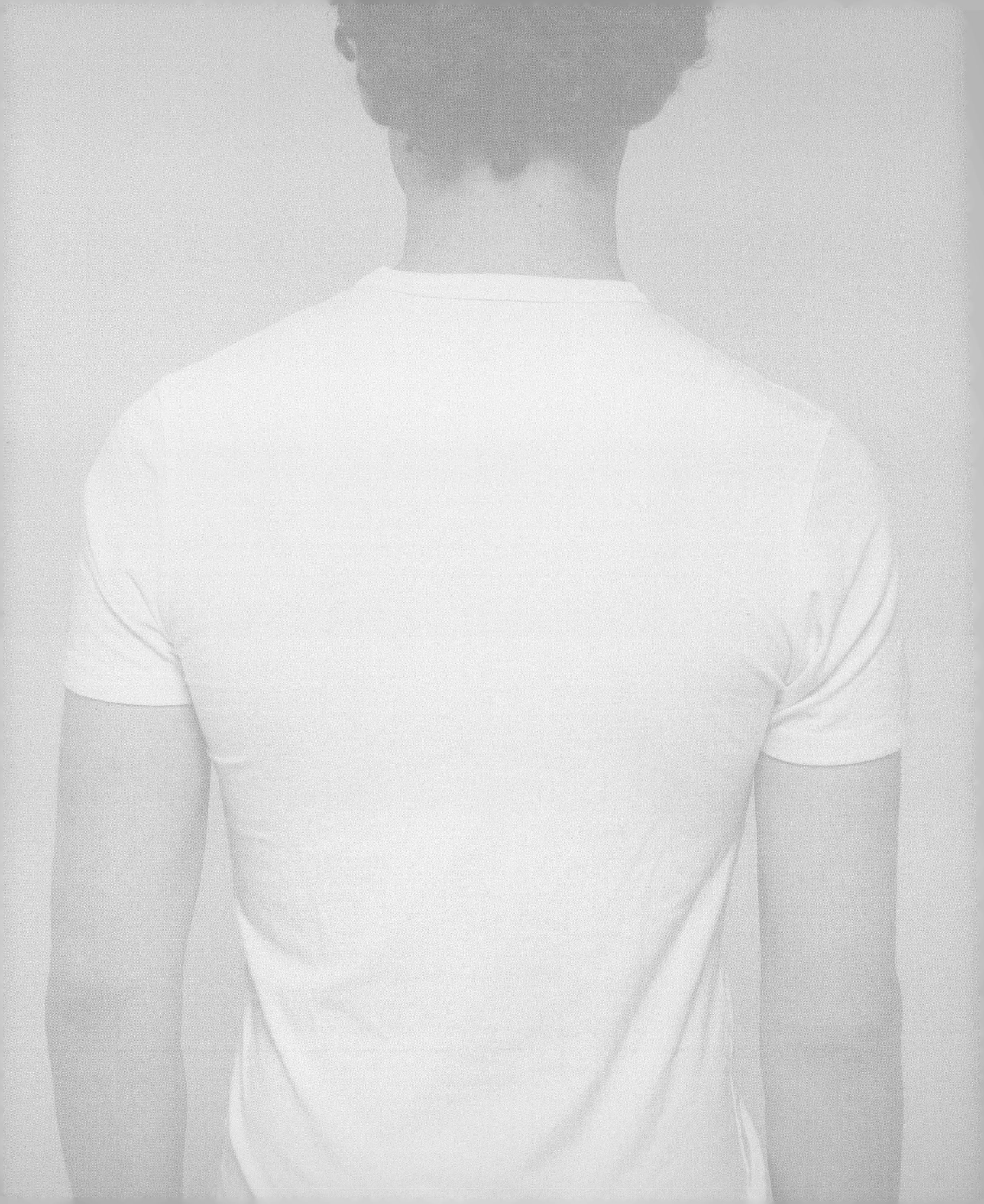

BACK PAIN – A SYMPTOM OF OUR LIFESTYLE

1

Pain

If you experience episodes of recurring back pain or suffer continuously from its debilitating effects, then I would like to offer you a quick word of encouragement. If the cause of your back pain is due to poor postural and tensional habits, there is a very good chance you can eliminate it from your life. And when I say you can eliminate it from your life, I really do mean *you*.

A visit to the doctor should initially be made to determine the cause of the pain and discomfort; in the unlikely situation that the pain is being caused by kidney problems or another serious condition it should be diagnosed quickly and appropriate treatment prescribed. This is important, and help should be sought without delay. However, if the cause of the pain is determined to be muscular and relating to posture, then can help yourself enormously.

Pain is the body's way of telling us that something is wrong. Just as a red warning light in the car it is there to be noticed and if we choose to ignore it, the cause may well develop into something more serious. However, we are all very different and while some people can experience severe and intolerable pain from an injury, cut or surgery, other people can find the same condition no worse than a mild irritation.

If we injure ourselves with a knife or prick ourselves on a thorn we experience sharp piercing pain; this is **acute pain**. We may apply antiseptic cream and bandage the wound, and if our body heals normally the pain will diminish over a few days or weeks and the wound will heal. If we over-use our muscles doing a work-out or excessive DIY or sport we may experience pain as a severe ache. A pulled muscle due to inappropriate bending, stretching or exercise will also cause a sharp acute pain which should diminish over a few days.

Chronic pain is quite different in that it lingers beyond an initial period. Views vary as to whether acute pain becomes

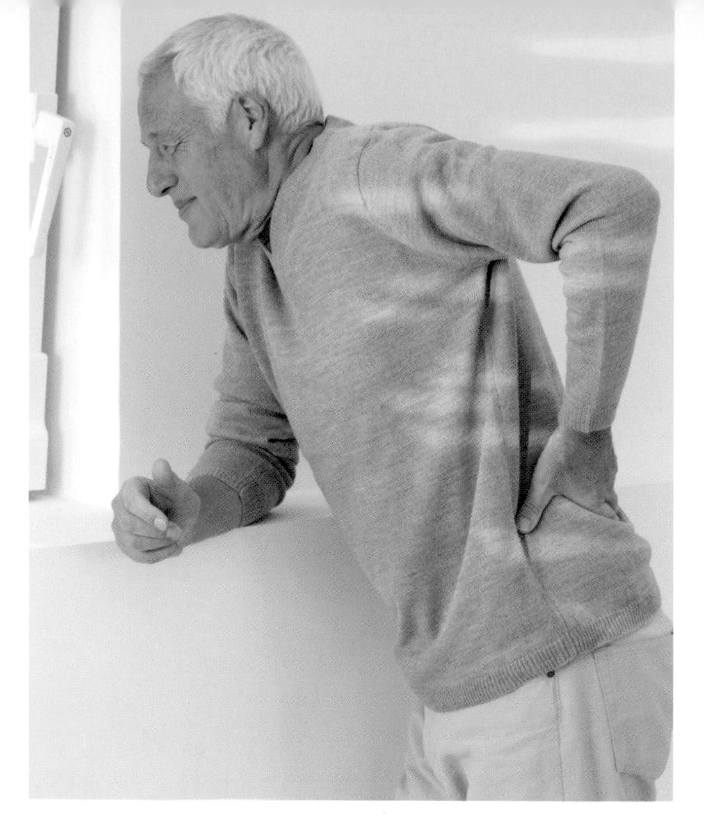

Back pain can be very debilitating and cause us to tense our whole body.

chronic after thirty days, three months or six months. However it is agreed that chronic pain lasts longer than an acute pain that heals relatively quickly. Chronic pain may be experienced as a dull ache or nagging diffused pain, which is rather more difficult to pinpoint and can be very tiring and wearing. The exact cause may not be easily diagnosed; X-rays, MRI and CT scans may not indicate the cause although, in the case of backache, they may show distortion to the spine and inter-vertebral discs. It is thought that chronic pain can be psychosomatic and emotional; our nervous system sends out warning signals to our brain which we feel as pain, but it can go into overdrive and produce more signals than the damage or injury may justify, so the level of pain we experience may be disproportionate to the actual situation.

Acute-on-chronic (or sub-acute) pain could be used to describe repeated episodes of back pain for several months. If you have experienced a prolonged bout of back pain which has caused you to become inactive, your muscles may become tender or stiff. Alexander Technique will be helpful to you as it promotes a lengthening and widening of stature which boosts blood and lymphatic circulation and decreases muscle stiffness.

How the brain feels pain

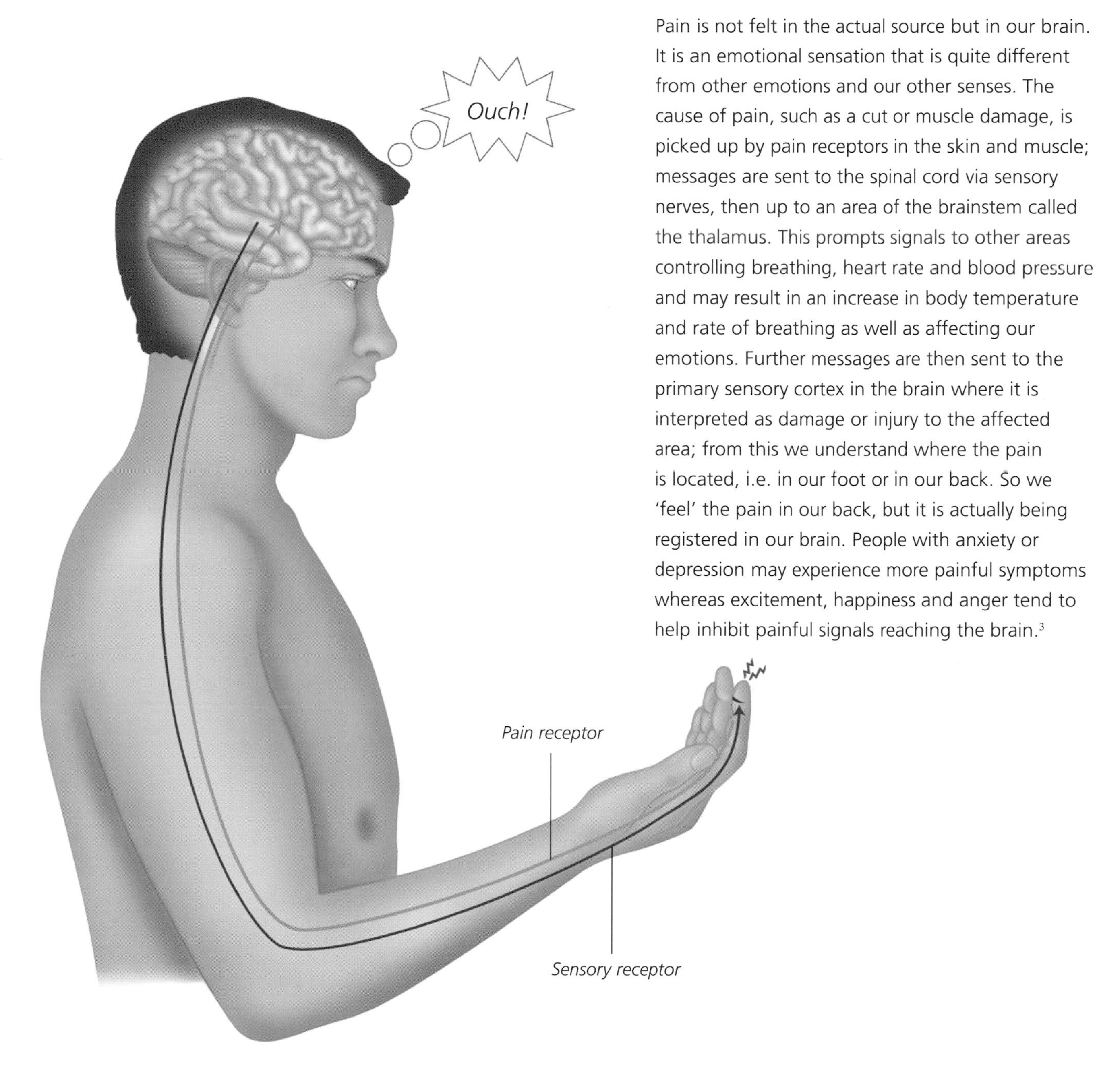

Pain is 'felt' in our brain, not at the source.

Pain is not felt in the actual source but in our brain. It is an emotional sensation that is quite different from other emotions and our other senses. The cause of pain, such as a cut or muscle damage, is picked up by pain receptors in the skin and muscle; messages are sent to the spinal cord via sensory nerves, then up to an area of the brainstem called the thalamus. This prompts signals to other areas controlling breathing, heart rate and blood pressure and may result in an increase in body temperature and rate of breathing as well as affecting our emotions. Further messages are then sent to the primary sensory cortex in the brain where it is interpreted as damage or injury to the affected area; from this we understand where the pain is located, i.e. in our foot or in our back. So we 'feel' the pain in our back, but it is actually being registered in our brain. People with anxiety or depression may experience more painful symptoms whereas excitement, happiness and anger tend to help inhibit painful signals reaching the brain.[3]

Causes of back pain

There are a great many causes of back pain, too numerous and complex to be covered in a book of this nature; however, the following examples will indicate some general 'injuries' or situations that can cause pain. While these examples may describe the cause of the painful symptom they are not the actual cause of the problem that needs to be addressed. This book will go on to address the reasons why most situations of back pain are related to posture and how we can avoid it.

Lactic acid is a by-product of any muscle activity but can build up in some muscles to cause tenderness and pain when the muscles are over-exercised. The lactic acid is normally dissipated when the muscles are rested but if we are stiffening our muscles through habit, or to protect ourselves against pain, this may not happen and the pain persists. This is because our body produces excessive amounts of lactic acid which can cause more pain as well as increased levels of anxiety and stress. This in turn causes us to stiffen more so we create even more lactic acid. Using the Alexander Technique helps us break through this cycle by releasing unnecessary tension, lengthening and widening and encouraging better circulation and breathing.

Muscle strain happens easily by excessive and unaccustomed muscular activity when the muscle is torn. The muscle fibre can be torn from the tendon causing the muscle to go into spasm, fill with blood and produce swelling. It can take several weeks or months to completely heal as long as the condition is not exacerbated. A doctor should be consulted and a regime of gentle exercise may be recommended to help blood circulation to the area to aid healing. However care and attention to one's poise by means of using the Alexander Technique will more than likely aid recovery.

Disc protrusion is where the inter-vertebral discs have been squashed by excessive and possibly continuous muscle tension around the spine. In such cases a distortion to the spinal curves is likely to show up in a scan and the disc will be bulging where its space has been reduced.

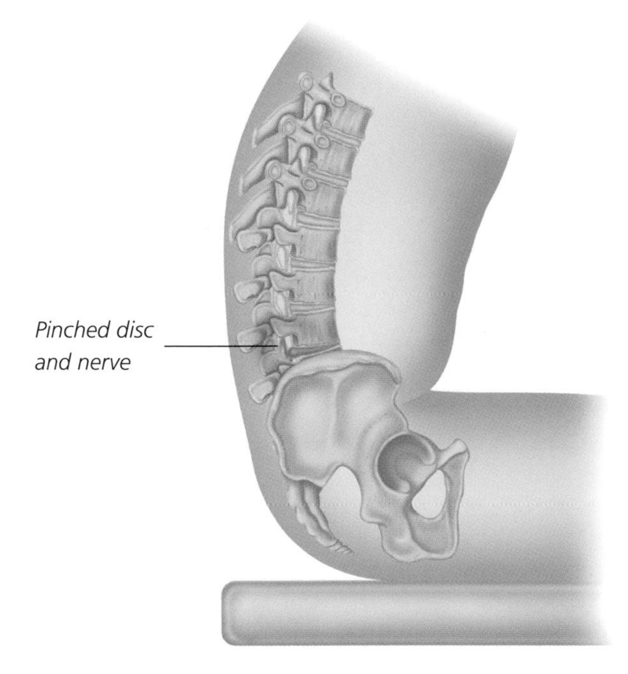

Slouching reverses the lumbar curve, compressing discs and putting pressure on nerves.

Prolapsed disc is often referred to as herniated or slipped disc and usually occurs in the lumbar spine. It is where the soft rubbery fluid normally contained within the fibrous walls of the disc has burst through the outer wall. This can put pressure on nerves leaving the spinal cord and can be very painful. It is understood that if the compressed disc is allowed to expand and return to its normal size very soon after the hernia, the fluid can return to within the disc so the pain diminishes and a healthy condition returns. However if the compression to the spine continues for any length of time, the disc's internal fluid can harden and become firm. In such cases surgery may be recommended to trim the disc.

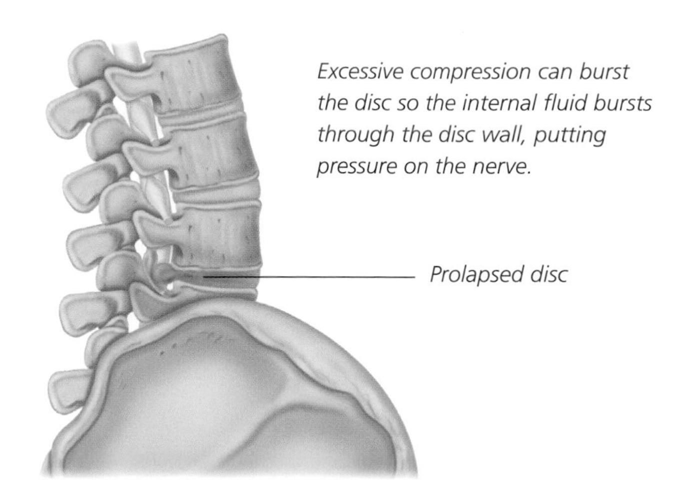

Excessive compression can burst the disc so the internal fluid bursts through the disc wall, putting pressure on the nerve.

Collapsed vertebrae is a condition usually associated with old age that can result from a combination of osteoporosis (a disease that thins and weakens the bones) coupled with a lifetime of poor posture and excessive downward pressure on the spine. Injury may also be an influence. Under such conditions the actual vertebrae of the spine that are intended to take the weight of the body can crumble.

Collapsed vertebrae

Normal vertebrae

Vertebrae can collapse with age when under long-term, excessive pressure.

Undiagnosed causes of pain are common. While the above causes of back pain may be diagnosed by a doctor, the majority of instances of back pain go undiagnosed. These are situations where the back may be under strain or muscles are in spasm or being used excessively in an unnatural manner, as part of our habitual way of sitting, standing and walking. X-rays may indicate excessive curvature to the spine, but this is not the reason for the pain, only an outcome of our muscular co-ordination. There may be nothing structurally wrong with our back but nevertheless we feel pain and discomfort in the upper, middle or lower back and possibly in the neck area. Such situations are usually triggered by a loss of natural poise and the onset of poor postural habits. The different ways of tensing and holding ourselves are infinite and it is impossible to describe every situation here, but there are some very common tendencies.

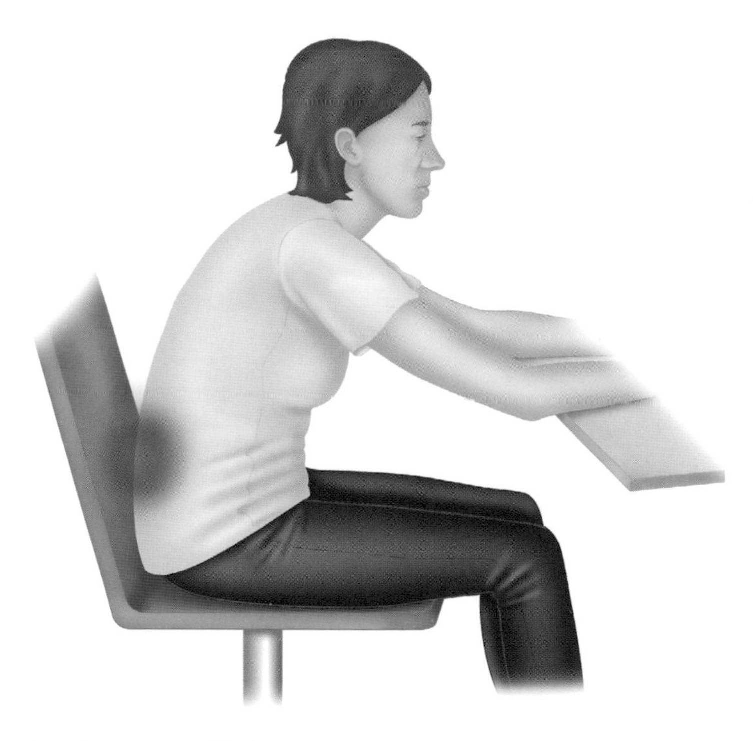

Slumping puts us off balance and causes strain and spinal compression.

Neck pain

The weight of our head can cause muscular strain to the neck and shoulders if it is not in good balance. Excessive stiffness and strain in the neck muscles can cause the cervical spine to become distorted and compress discs. This puts pressure on nerves which may also send painful symptoms down our arms causing numbness or nerve tingling as well as headaches. Having a free neck with good head balance is fundamental to healthy poise. The relationship between our head, neck and back determines how our whole body functions. The Alexander Technique will help enable you to free your neck from unnecessary tension and restore natural, upright, balanced poise without strain. Neck and shoulder tension is associated with the 'fight-or-flight reflex' (see page 22).

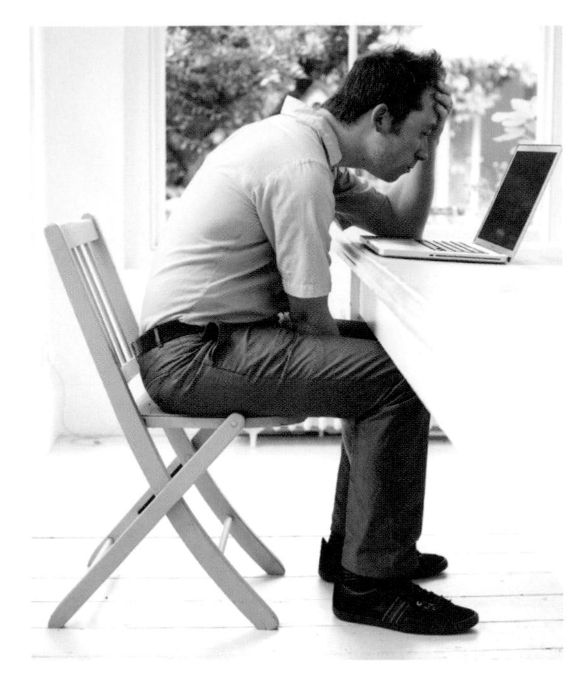

Slouching unbalances us, putting our neck and back under strain.

Upper back pain

This is often linked with neck pain and occurs when we shorten our natural height by stooping downward, rounding our shoulders or slumping over a desk or computer. The thoracic spine can become excessively rounded (known as kyphosis), and our head may jut forward from our body rather than being poised in balance over our shoulders. If this type of position is held for long periods of time, muscles can become over-developed and constantly contracted; discs also become distorted and compressed. Hunched shoulders can also cause tension around the neck and upper back. A tendency to drop our neck and head forward puts a lot of pressure on the seventh vertebra, putting the surrounding muscles under significant and unhealthy strain.

A different type of problem can be caused by over-straightening the thoracic spine, as can be encouraged in some forms of dance. This too is a distortion of the spine that needs to be addressed with the overall poise of the individual.

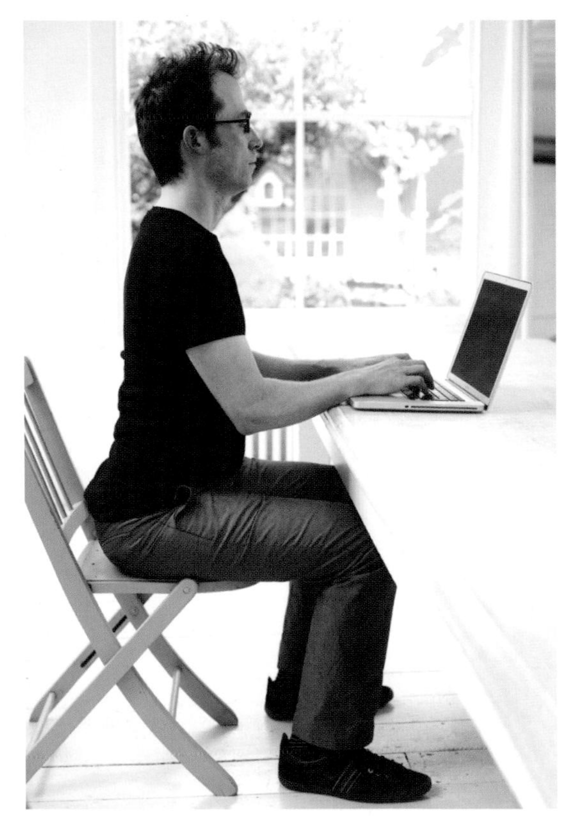

Over-arching the lower back and stiffening.

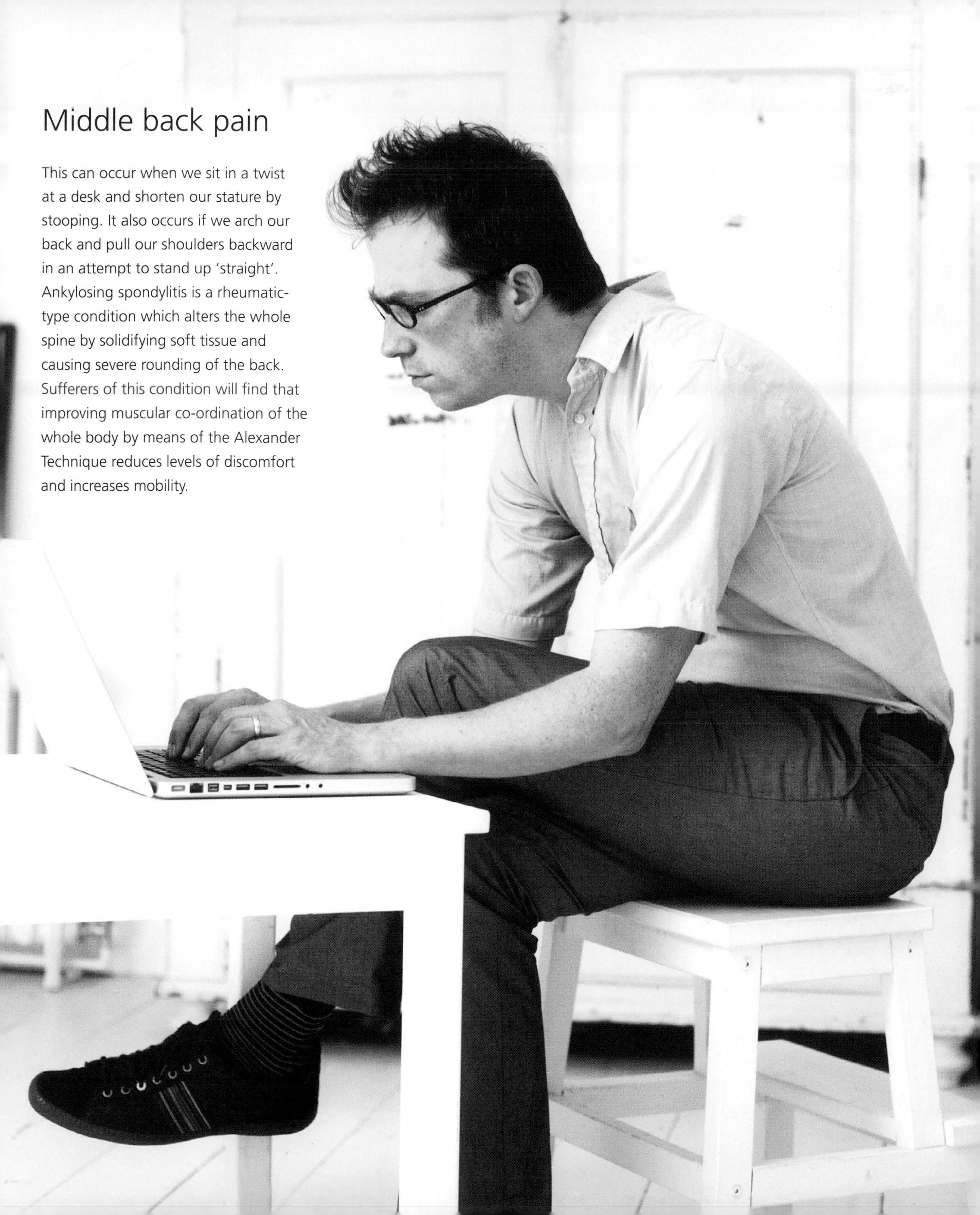

Middle back pain

This can occur when we sit in a twist at a desk and shorten our stature by stooping. It also occurs if we arch our back and pull our shoulders backward in an attempt to stand up 'straight'. Ankylosing spondylitis is a rheumatic-type condition which alters the whole spine by solidifying soft tissue and causing severe rounding of the back. Sufferers of this condition will find that improving muscular co-ordination of the whole body by means of the Alexander Technique reduces levels of discomfort and increases mobility.

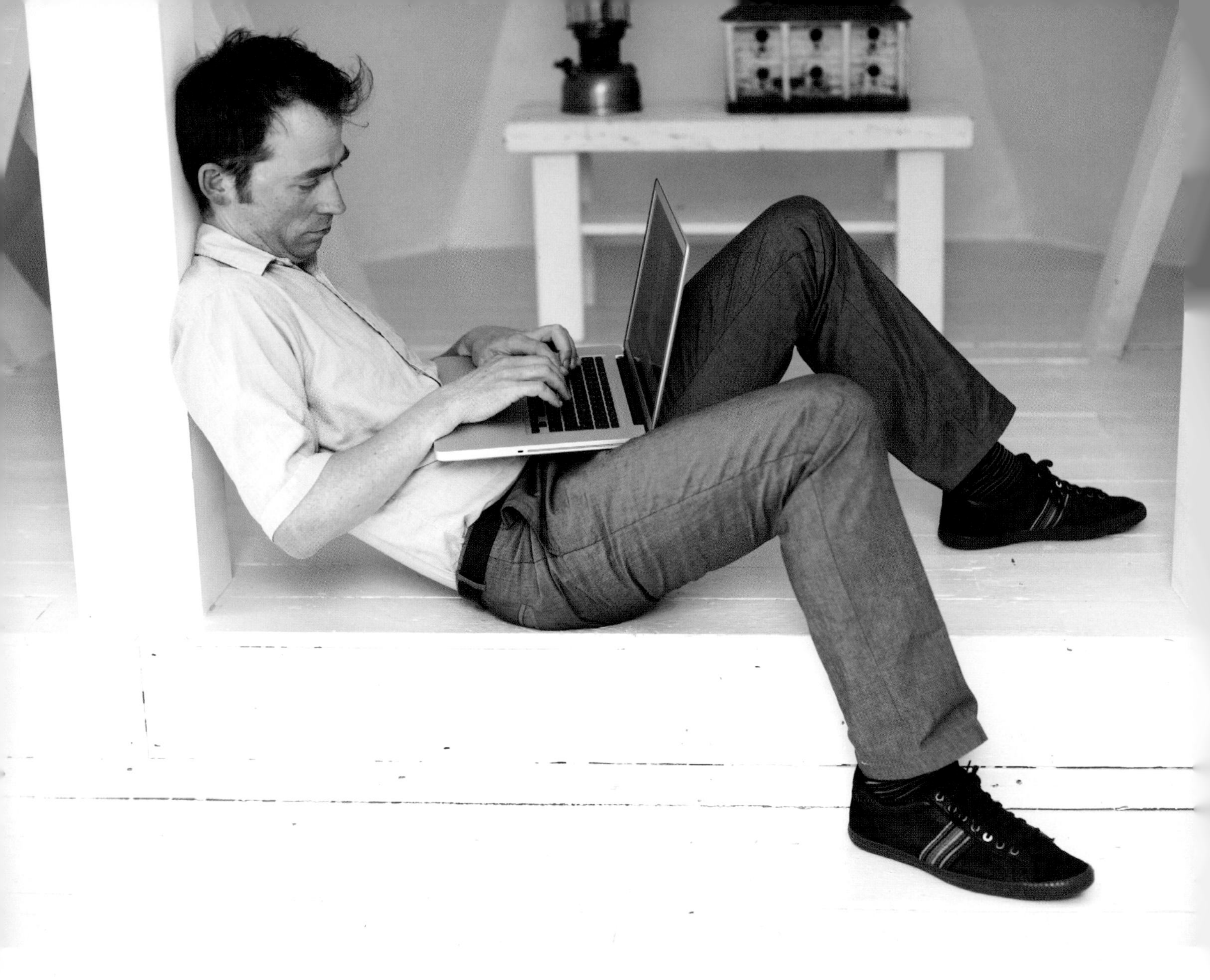

Lower back pain

Lower back pain or lumbago is by far the most common form of back pain. The lumbar curve in our lower back plays an important role in supporting our body in a balanced way while also providing flexibility to the spine. If this curve is lost or inverted a great deal of extra pressure is put onto the discs and surrounding muscles can become excessively tense. Pain in the lower back can be caused by slumping in a chair, or sitting with legs crossed or in a twist. It can also be caused by over-reaching to pick something up. If our body is not in good balance this can result in a torn muscle. Lumbar pain can also be caused by over-arching the lumbar spine (lordosis) when standing or sitting. This 'narrowing' of the back tilts the pelvis, causing our abdominal organs to 'spill' forward and our tummy to protrude, increasing the strain on the back. If poise is not addressed this can lead to a prolapsed disc.

Collapsing our stature puts pressure on internal organs and sacrum.

Pain in the sacrum

This can be caused by the sacro-iliac joint being slightly out of alignment. The sacrum forms both part of our spine and also the pelvis and is held in position by very strong tissue. If we twist awkwardly and vigorously we can put our sacrum very slightly out of alignment so the surrounding muscles go into spasm. An osteopathic adjustment may help to restore a healthy situation. However, if this is a recurring problem it is likely to be associated with postural habits that need to be addressed.

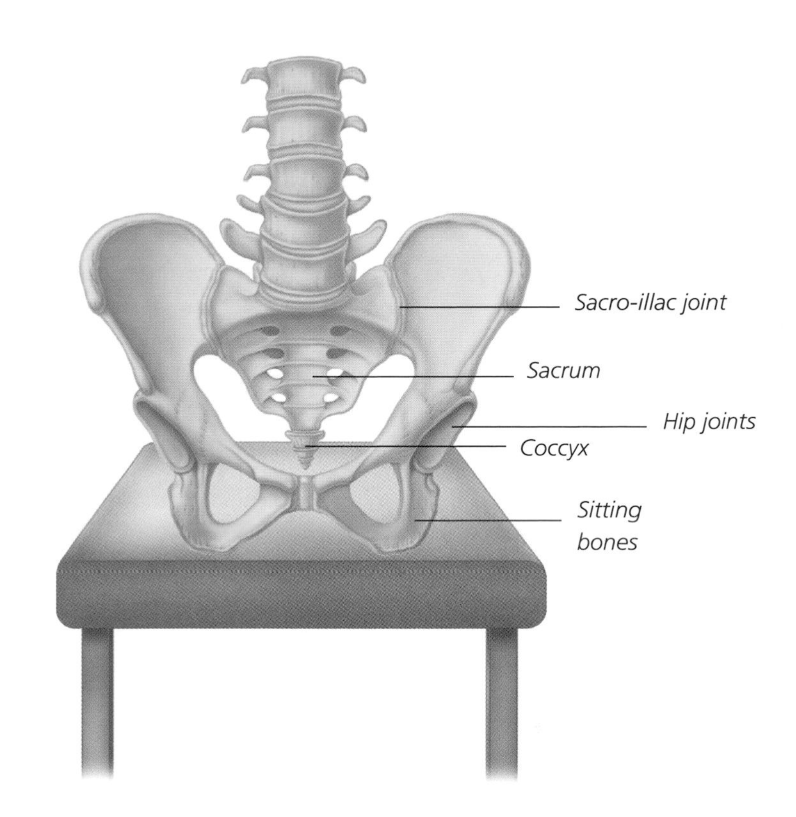

Pain in the coccyx

The coccyx is a small group of 5–6 bones located underneath the sacrum, rather like a tail. The coccyx has pelvic muscle attachments which, if they go into spasm, can cause pain in the pelvic floor or thighs. There are various causes of coccyx pain (or coccydynia), many being postural. Some people may have a longer coccyx than usual and if the tendency is to sit with the pelvis out of balance, pressure may be put onto the coccyx by a hard seat. Postural re-training can help muscles to release unnecessary tension, thus benefiting the pelvic floor, legs and back. Bruising to the coccyx may take some time to disappear once the cause has been rectified, but improved 'use' helps to avoid aggravation so it can heal more quickly.

In the majority of the above situations (that have been generalised for expediency) the cause of pain is likely to be associated with poor posture and can therefore be helped by restoring healthy balanced and upright poise.

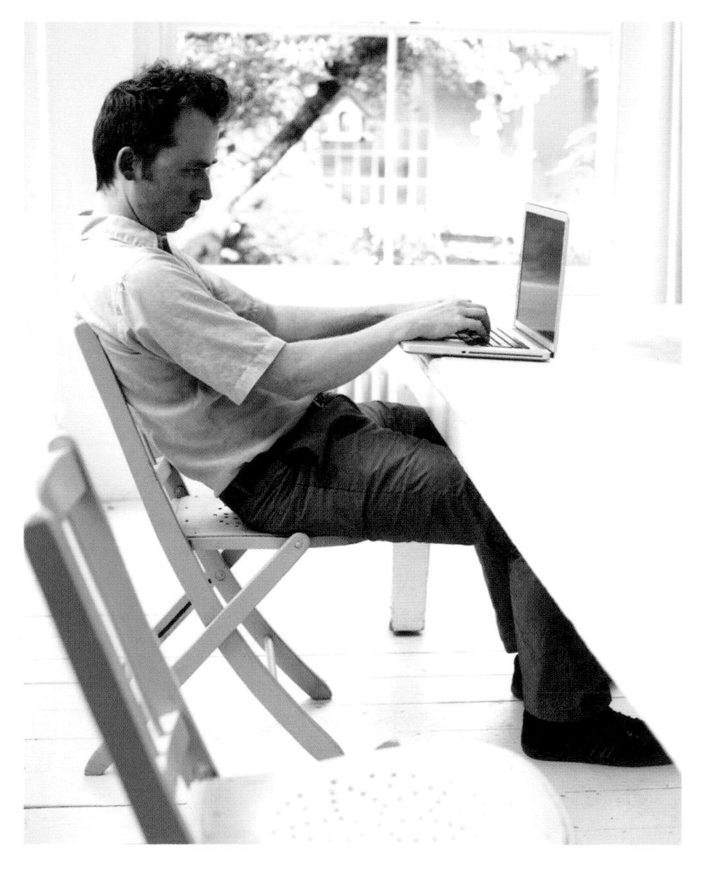

Slumping puts pressure on lower back, sacrum and neck.

Emotions and pain

Emotions are an intrinsic part of the whole body. There is evidence that increased stress, depression or anger can heighten our sense of pain, whereas positive emotions such as happiness, joy and excitement can inhibit the passing of painful symptoms to the brain so we experience less discomfort.[4]

Prolonged bouts of back pain can become very wearing and prevent us from sleeping or enjoying ourselves to the full. They can also cause depression, irrational anger and even emotional friction in relationships, affecting the quality of our home life.

The Alexander Technique helps bring about a quality of expansiveness which can lift our spirits as though a load has been taken from us. Lessons in the technique not only help eliminate the co-ordinational causes of back pain but can also lighten our mood.

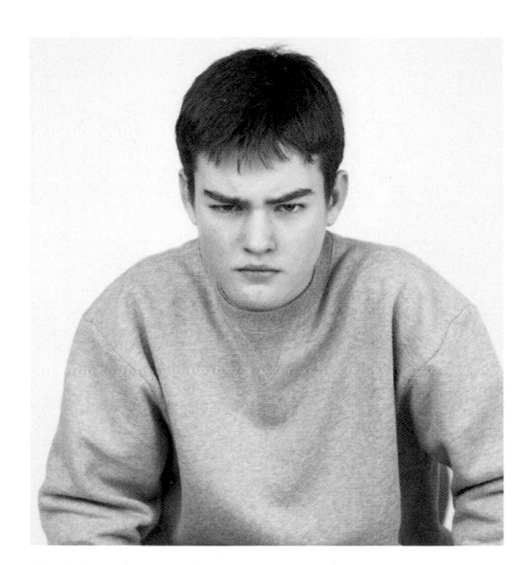

Back pain can be very wearing, causing stress and anger.

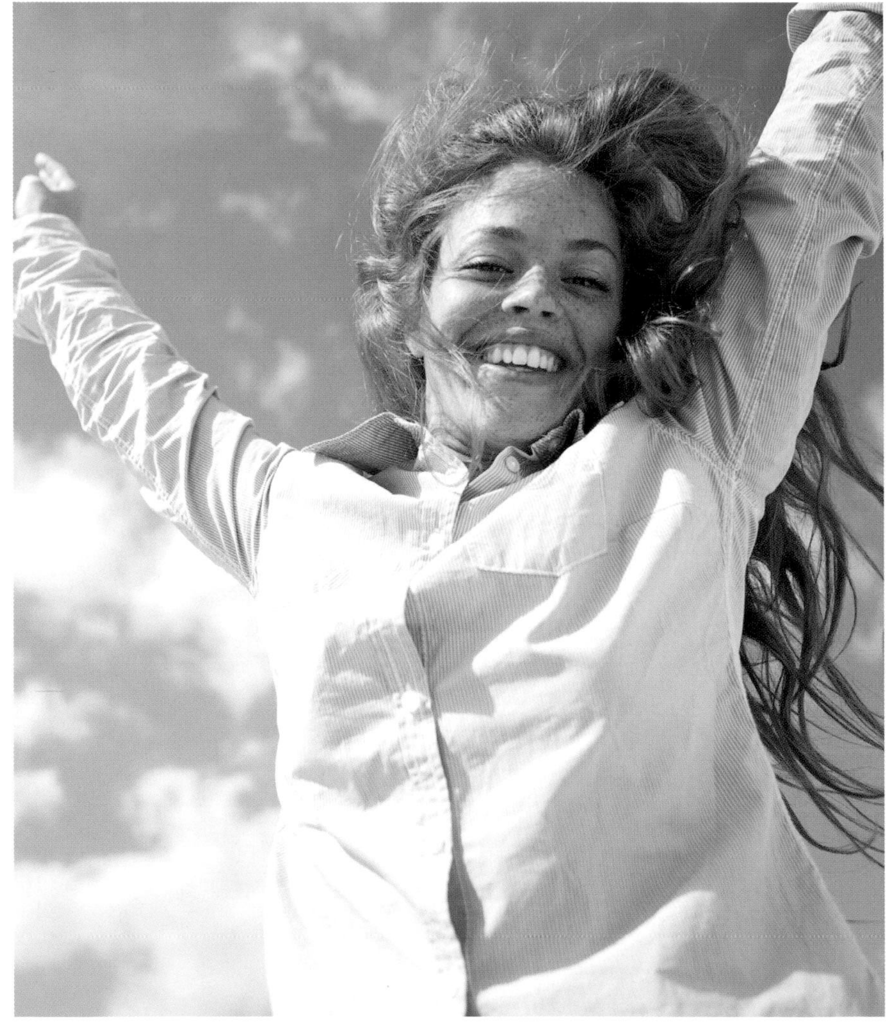

Releasing tension makes us more expansive and can lift our mood.

Enjoying life more fully

Someone said to me a while ago that her husband is so much easier to live with since he started having lessons in the Alexander Technique! Well, I wouldn't have known if he was good or bad to live with, but how this might be is understandable if we consider that with a reduction in tension, an improved physical balance and expansive stature come emotional centredness and calmness; the two go hand in hand. It helps us be happy and more fun.

Relief from pain can lift our spirits and we may no longer shy away from social situations but enter into them with far more enthusiasm. Improvements to our poise can lead to reduced physical tensions and emotional stress; we can become more easy-going and tolerant. With the Alexander Technique we become more physically balanced and may feel more emotionally centred too; this helps our confidence and security. By learning the Alexander Technique, we may not only change our own life, but also benefit the lives of those around us.

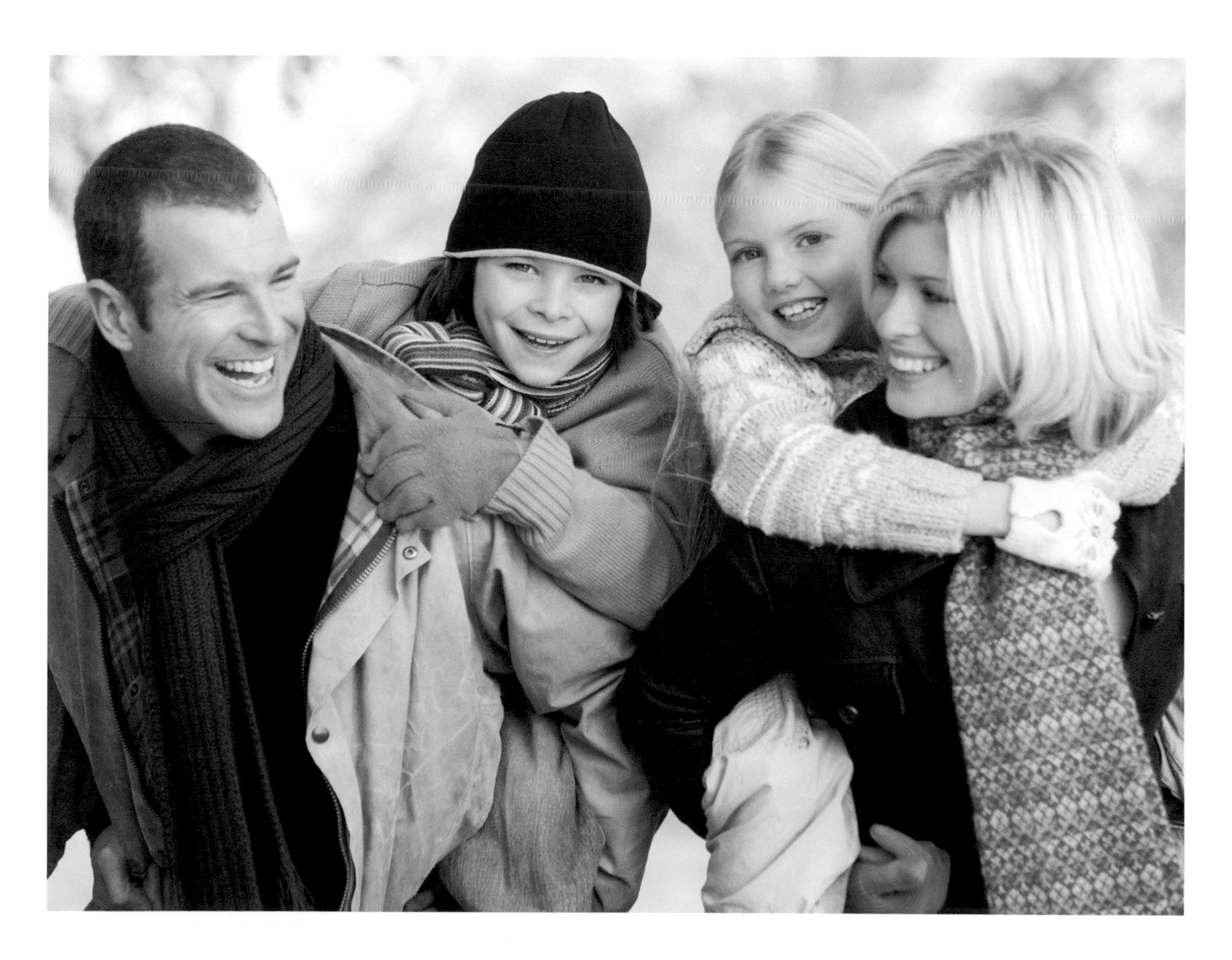

Fight-or-flight response

Often referred to as the 'startle pattern', our response to life-threatening situations enables us to escape from and deal with danger. However, this instinctive reaction can also become habitual if constantly repeated, with serious health consequences. Along with an increase in breathing rate, circulation and adrenalin, the pattern prepares us to handle danger by shortening our stature so we become smaller, pushing our head forward, hunching our shoulders, stiffening our arms and flexing our legs. Any fearful situation, such as being reprimanded at school or facing the boss in difficult circumstances for instance, puts us momentarily into this pattern to a greater or lesser degree, and this can become habitual. Many of us display some aspects of the pattern in our everyday posture, causing unnecessary and constant strain, imbalance and wear and tear on our body. With the improved awareness and conscious control that the Alexander Technique gives us we can unlearn the habits, thus restoring natural poise and calm.

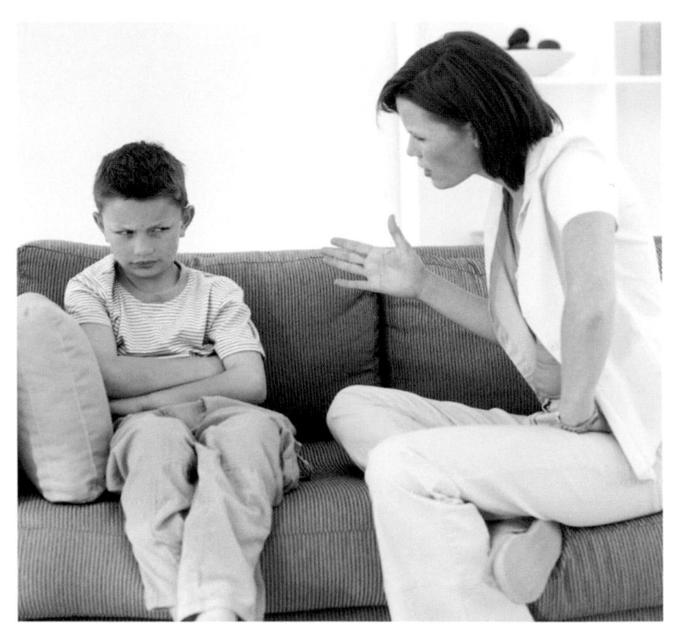

Fearful situations put us into startle pattern.

The 'startle pattern' is initiated by stiffening of the neck muscles and displacement of the head followed by other reactions to the torso, arms and legs. The fixed and imbalanced position of the head upsets the balance and co-ordination of our whole body, putting our back under increased strain. However, if we learn to 'inhibit' the neck tensions, we can successfully reduce our reaction and prevent overall startle pattern. We can then maintain free upright poise and regular breathing, and avoid putting ourselves into such a high state of alert, so remaining calm.

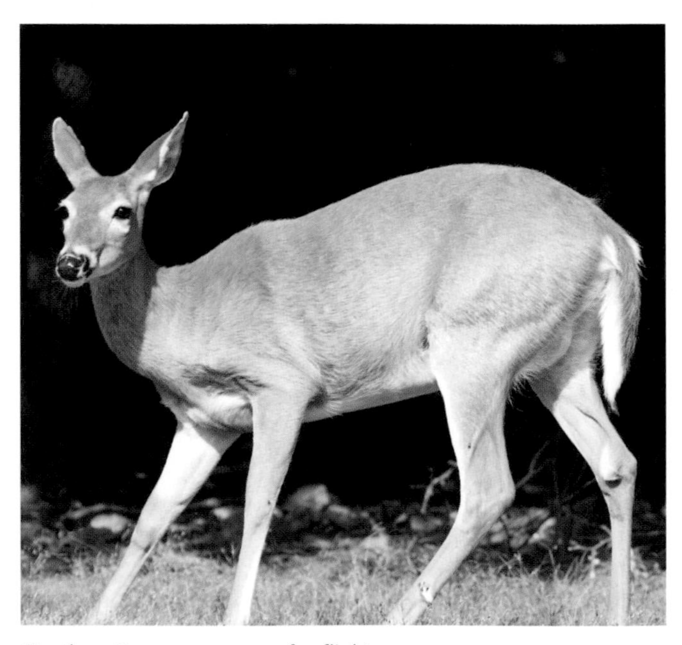

Startle pattern prepares us for flight.

Movement to help circulation and repair damaged tissue

If we are injured or experiencing pain our body tends to stiffen as a means of stabilising and protecting the damaged area. We may even make guarded movements as part of pain-avoidance behaviour, stiffening our body to minimise or avoid discomfort. However this does not help the healing process as muscle tension tends to restrict blood circulation, inhibiting the amount of fresh oxygenated blood reaching the injury. Releasing muscular tension by using the Alexander Technique will not only improve poise and circulation but will also free up our breathing mechanism (see Chapter 6), further enabling the oxygenation of the blood.

Gentle exercise such as stretching will also help to promote healing as the lengthening muscles will improve blood circulation. Aerobic activities, such as walking or gentle swimming, increase the heart rate and blood circulation so we are breathing faster and more deeply; this will also raise endorphin levels so we feel happier. High impact exercise, such as football or jogging, will also increase heart rates and blood circulation but may cause further injury or exacerbate the existing condition. If we are in pain, exercise should be restricted to gentle aerobic activities and built up slowly as our improving condition permits.

By learning the Alexander Technique as outlined in this book you will change the functioning of your body, increase blood circulation and oxygenation, reduce pain, increase endorphin levels and improve your sense of happiness and well-being.

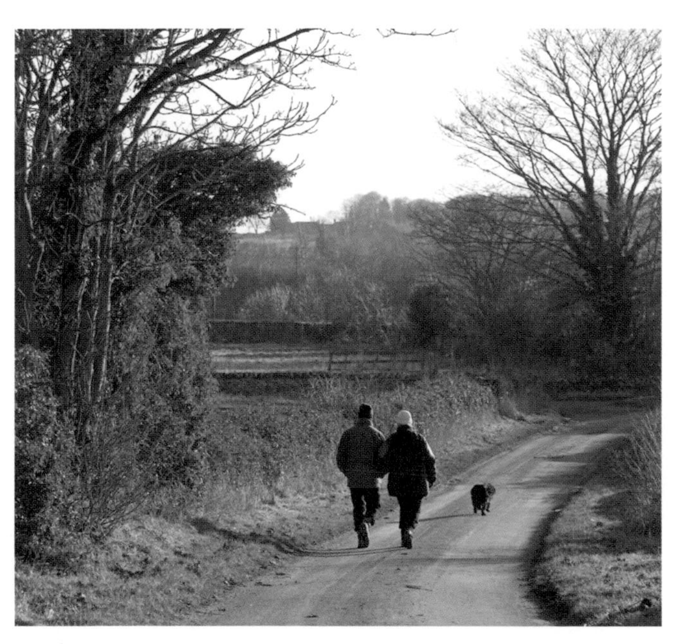

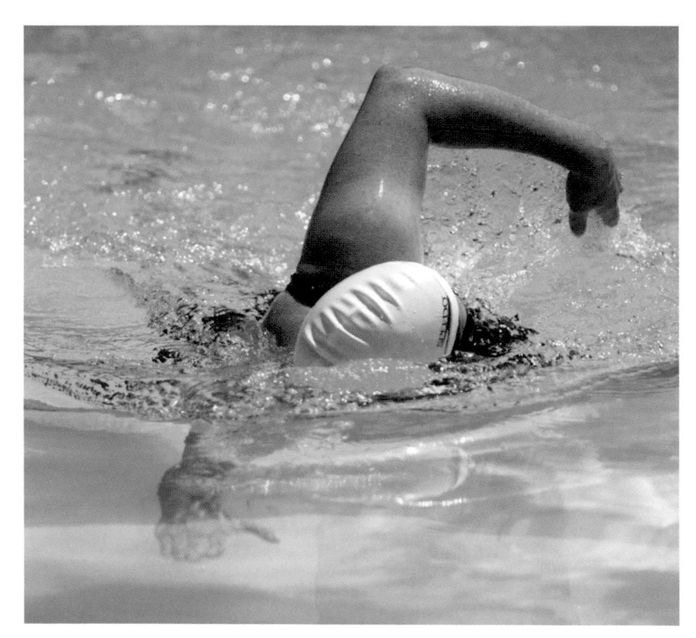

Gentle exercise promotes increased blood circulation and healing.

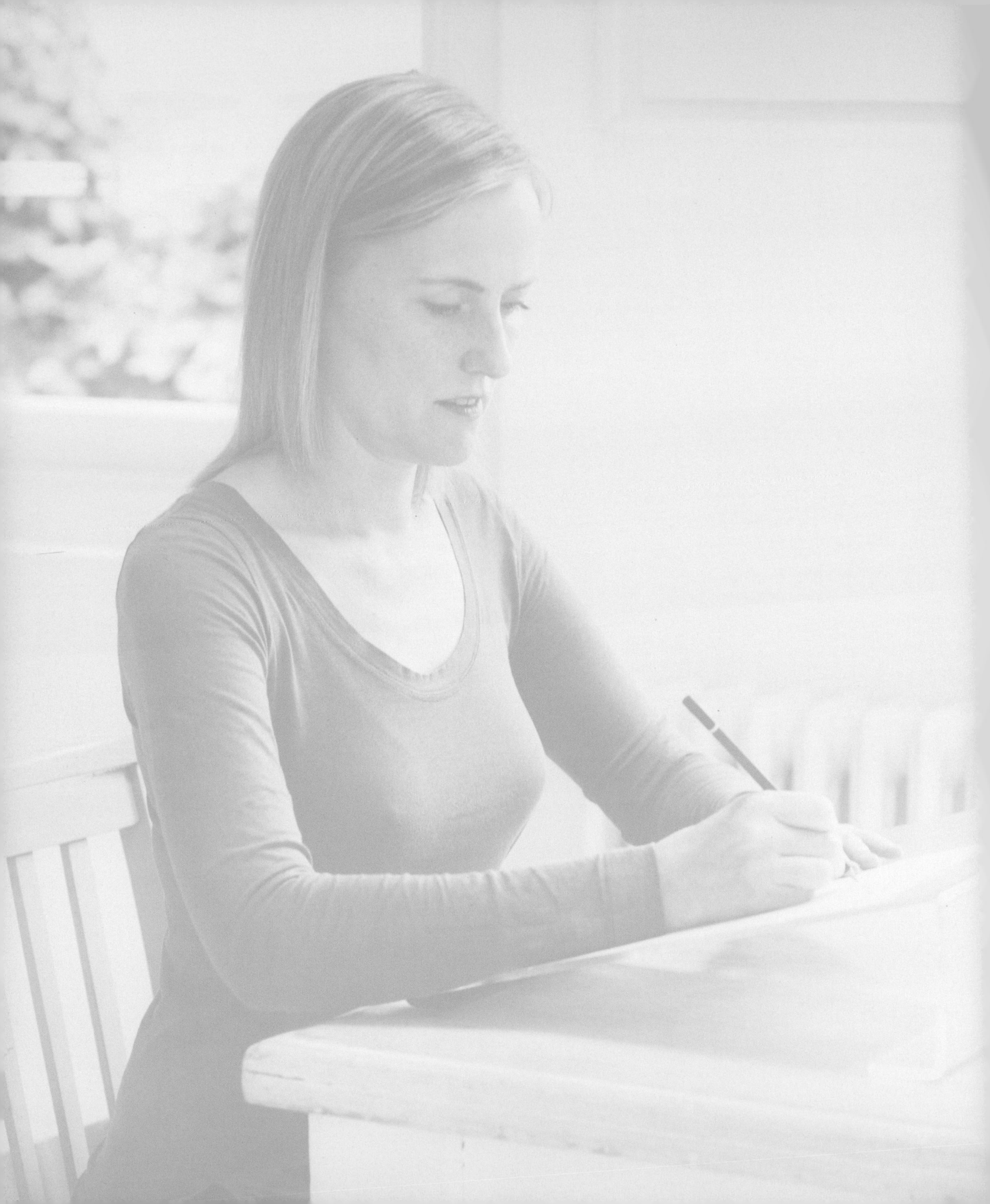

WHY GOOD POISE IS IMPORTANT

2

How we have evolved

Good posture is not a textbook ideal but a necessity for healthy living, and back pain is a clear signal that all is not right. As with any piece of machinery or equipment, our body needs to be used properly for it to give long-lasting service without breaking down or deteriorating before its time. If we consider how we drive a car, it's important to change gear by using the clutch otherwise we will damage the gearbox, and if we want to move forward, we release the handbrake so as not to inhibit forward motion and wear out the brake pads. As humans we are bio-mechanical and our mechanisms of movement must be used in accordance with our design in order for them to work efficiently. This means being in balance, expanding to our full height and stature to take the pressure off our joints and moving with minimal effort.

Any equipment needs to be used appropriately for it to give long lasting service. Humans are no different.

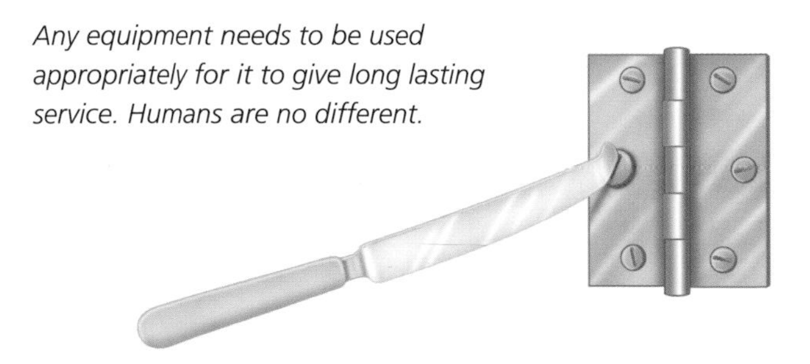

There are a great many obvious differences between humans and other vertebrate mammals such as dogs, cats, horses, cheetahs, sheep and squirrels. First, they have four legs and we have two; they do not sit at a desk for ten hours a day, drive cars, cycle, wear high heels, carry shoulder bags or feign a cultured stoop to look 'cool'. They're far too sensible for that! One of the biggest differences between humans and other vertebrate mammals is the size of our brain and our ability to make choices. Our intelligence sets us apart from other creatures.

Over millions of years we have evolved as a species, from the amphibians that originally came onto land, developing into four-legged creatures through various stages of evolution to become rather ape-like using long arms to walk and run. Gradually these creatures evolved into the primate family Hominidae within which there were many variants or sub-species. Anatomically modern humans (Homo sapiens) first appear in the fossil record in Africa about 195,000 years ago and co-existed in some parts of the world with other hominid species such as Homo neanderthalensis until as recently as 30,000 years ago.

It is by no accident that primitive humans began to walk as bipeds. Being on two feet was helpful for wading through deep water and reaching upward into the trees for fruit. No longer needing arms and hands to help them balance, the upper limbs became shorter and lighter to carry around.

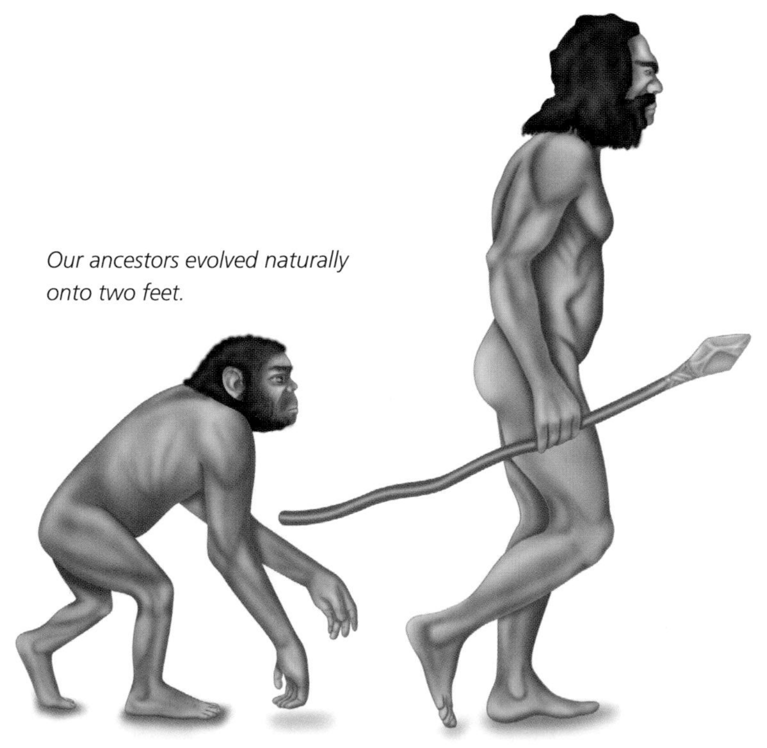

Our ancestors evolved naturally onto two feet.

Evidence shows that our psycho-physical organism evolved over millennia; the vestibular mechanism in our inner ear rotated through 90 degrees enabling us to develop from a four-legged creature to a two-legged biped and maintain balance in an upright poise. Eventually we became upright Homo sapiens who now meet down at the pub, share an office and play tennis.

In relative terms, the history of the modern world is very short in comparison to the overall evolution of our species. Our ancestors who had evolved onto two feet were still running and hunting until just a few thousand years ago, after millions of years of evolution. Now here we are; you're sitting reading this book and we're not that dissimilar to our cavemen ancestors but our activities and lifestyle are dramatically different. We now perform a multitude of tasks, many of which are very repetitive, such as sitting at a desk, typing at keyboards and driving cars for long periods. We sit on chairs yet our ancestors sat on their haunches rather as Aborigines might still do today. Our body is really not very different from that of our ancestors who ran and hunted, however evolution has not caught up with the requirements of modern living.

Here we are using a physique which is arguably far better suited to an active lifestyle than today's sedentary lifestyle. It's no wonder we are prone to back pain if we do not take care of ourselves.

Homo sapiens have created a world and lifestyle that require quite a different physique in order to survive healthily. Yet, most of us do not use any of our advanced intelligence to help us cope physically and mentally with the modern environment. And while designers may come up with new styles of chairs, desks and equipment to help us, on an individual level most of us have no more awareness of how we move, sit or stand than early cavemen.

F.M. Alexander evolved a technique that provides us with a means of looking after ourselves from a postural and human-functioning point of view in any activity. His technique enables us to maintain healthy co-ordination and 'use' of our whole body and mind, so we can use our intelligence to help bring the best of ourselves to any task we undertake while also minimising postural problems and avoiding such debilitating conditions as backache.

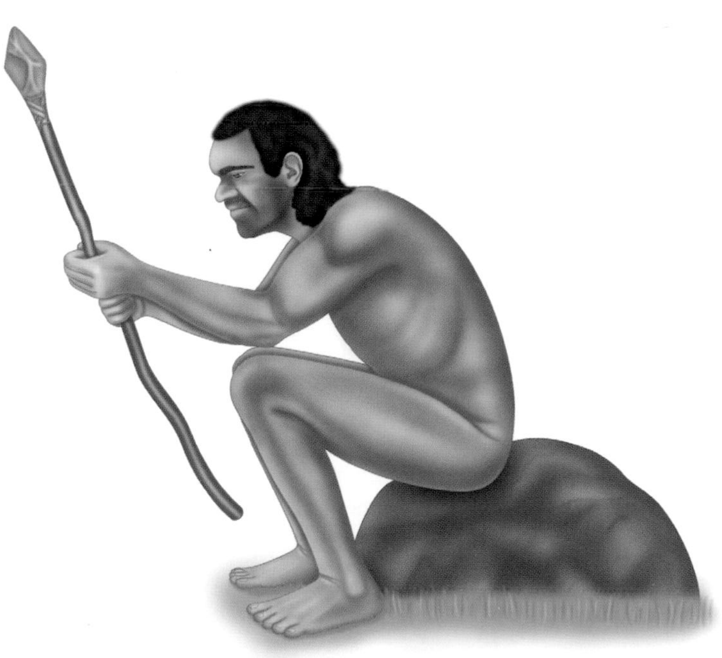

Most of us do not use any of our advanced intelligence to help us cope with our modern environment.

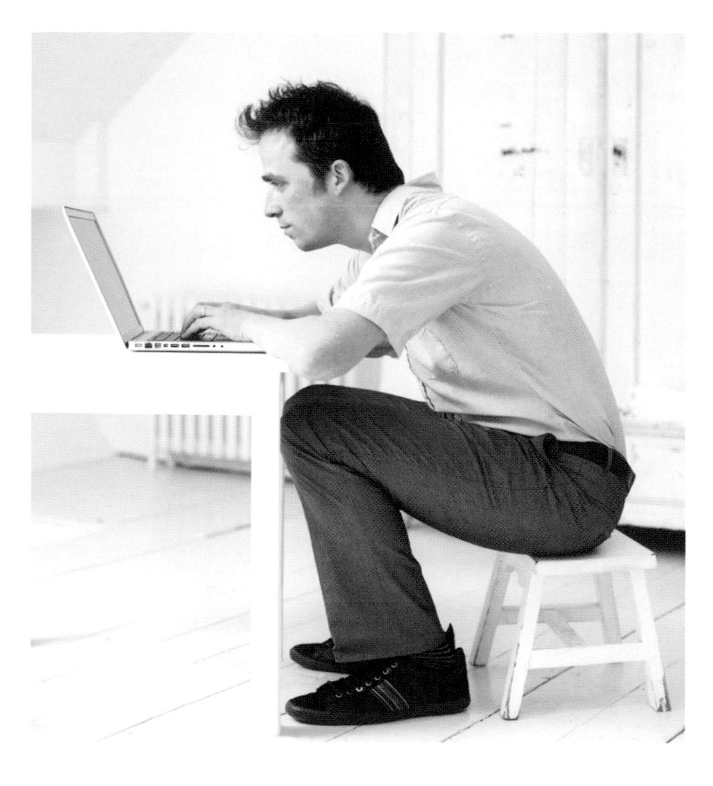

F.M. Alexander

Frederick Matthias Alexander was born in Winyard, southern Tasmania, on 20 January 1869, and lived with his seven siblings and parents on a large farm. He had respiratory problems from an early age but these improved by the time he was nine. He was a precocious child with a quick temper, but despite this developed an affinity with horses and a love of poetry that would last all his life. Financial problems at home forced him to seek a variety of jobs and his keen interest in theatre, particularly Shakespeare, took him to Melbourne where he continued his acting training.

He became a successful professional actor working in Sydney and Melbourne specialising in performing a one-man show that included poetry, excerpts from Shakespeare, drama and humour. However it was not long before he began to experience vocal problems, particularly hoarseness, during performances. Friends in the audience said they could hear him gasping for breath and sucking air through his mouth between phrases. Doctors and voice specialists advised him to rest and to use his voice as little as possible between performances, but within a short time of commencing the next performance he would become increasingly hoarse from projecting to large audiences. His hoarseness developed over time, eventually culminating in a complete loss of voice.

Before one very important engagement his doctors had said that complete rest beforehand for two weeks would ensure he would perform successfully without vocal problems. On the night of the performance he was completely free of hoarseness but before he was halfway through his programme his voice was in a terrible state; by the end of the evening he could barely speak.

Clearly the medical treatment and advice of his doctors to rest was not working. He confronted his doctor: 'Is it not fair to conclude that it was something I was doing that evening in using my voice that was the cause of trouble?' The doctor was in agreement but was unable to say precisely what was wrong, so Alexander replied: 'If that is so, I must try and find out for myself'.[5]

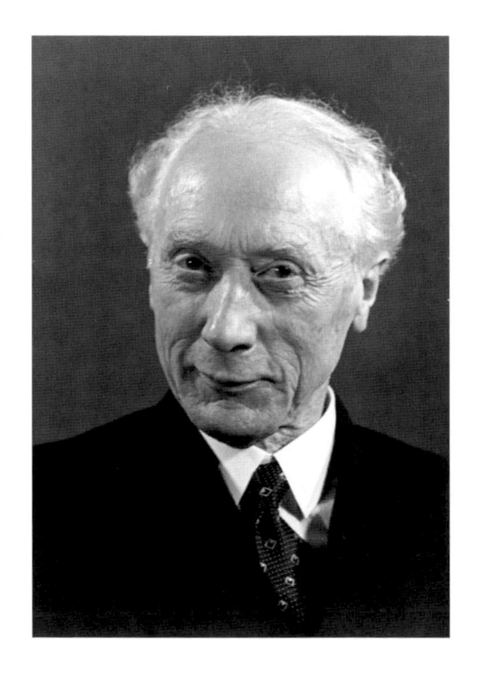

Determined that his vocal problems would not force him to retire from the stage, he set off on a long process of self-observation and examination, eventually concluding that it was the manner in which he spoke that was causing the problem.

With the aid of mirrors Alexander was able to observe how he used his body in the act of speaking both in ordinary speech and also when reciting. Very soon he noticed that while reciting he had a distinct tendency to pull back his head, depress his larynx and suck in breath through his mouth, things that were not obvious in normal speech but nevertheless existed to a lesser degree. On examination of his

F.M. Alexander giving a lesson.

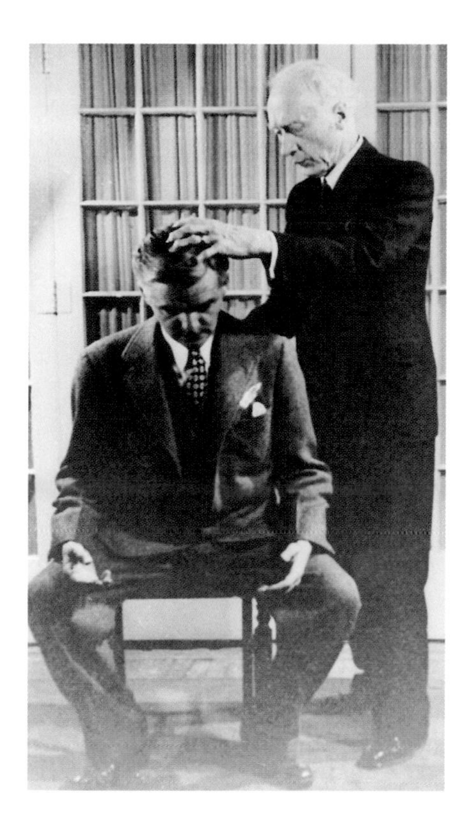

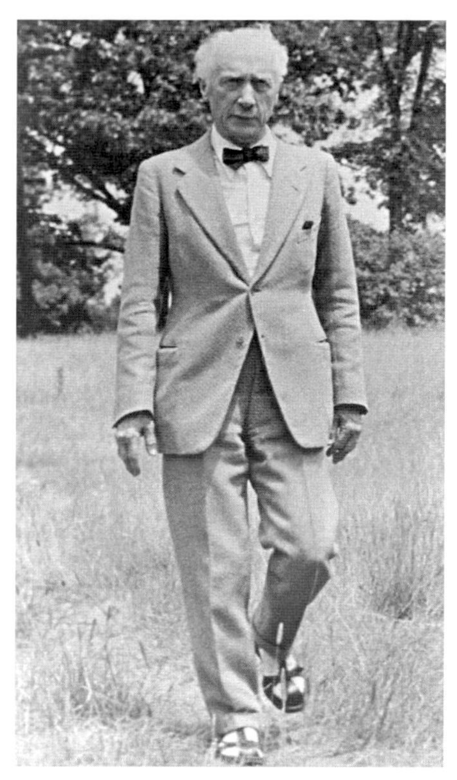

actions more closely, he further noticed that while reciting he braced his legs, arched his back and raised his chest, all of which he discovered interfered with his natural co-ordination and constituted a misuse of the working parts of his organism.

Alexander discovered that his tendency to retract his head caused a shortening of his spine, but if he allowed his head to roll forward naturally with the aid of gravity, the spine could naturally lengthen. In addition he noticed that every time he opened his mouth to speak he instinctively pulled his head backward and depressed his larynx. Alexander realised that preventing the wrong thing from happening was fundamental to making further progress. He went on to discover that if he inhibited an instant response to movement or speech, this gave him time to direct himself to lengthen in stature first rather than shorten and tense his neck. By stopping to think first, he could control how he spoke or performed any movement.

As he learnt to inhibit the harmful tendencies of retracting his head, depressing his larynx and thereby preventing the wrong 'use' of his body, he created healthy conditions which allowed the inflammation of his vocal cords and irritation to his mucous membrane to heal. Alexander's experimentation went on for many years, during which time he not only cured his vocal problems, but his whole stance changed as he came up to his full height and stature in the most natural and free manner. He was again able to perform on stage and other actors asked if he could show them his method. Alexander initially gained a reputation as the 'Breathing Man' and doctors referred patients to him with ailments such as asthma and bronchitis. But it was soon recognised that his technique helped to change the manner of 'use' of the whole self, to improve not only voice and breathing but also the efficient working of the whole body and mind, promoting good general health and well-being.

Eventually he was recommended to travel to London to meet a number of eminent doctors in order to demonstrate his technique. Alexander arrived in London in 1904 where he got to know a number of prominent people, including Aldous Huxley, George Bernard Shaw, Sir Charles Sherrington, Sir Stafford Cripps and Lord Lytton, who all advocated the benefits of Alexander's technique.

In 1930 Alexander was encouraged by several eminent doctors to set up a training course for teachers of his technique. He continued to instruct teachers on his three-year full-time training course until he died on 10 October 1955. Awareness of his technique has spread and there are now thousands of qualified teachers practising worldwide.

Alexander Technique: now and for a healthy future

Life is not about sitting around doing nothing, wrapping ourselves up in cotton wool and avoiding all movements and occupations that are potentially harmful. While we are in pain, naturally we will be taking great care to avoid straining or aggravating our discomfort, but we want to get beyond this stage. We want to be able to engage in all sorts of activities and start living our life to the full again. And there is every chance that we can.

The Alexander Technique is a practical means of helping us maintain good poise, no matter what our activity. Unlike treatments or therapies that may give special exercises to overcome a problem, it's a self-help method that we learn to use throughout the day, while we are doing all the things we enjoy doing. We can benefit from 'using' the Alexander Technique while engaging in a range of activities from walking, bending, sitting, reading, working on the computer or watching television, to answering the phone, doing the ironing, gardening or playing sport.

By looking after ourselves now we help to create postural conditions that enable our body to function healthily, move around free of pain and, where we can, engage in activities that make us happy and fulfilled. By doing this we not only improve our quality of life today, but safeguard our future so we can live healthier for longer. It's an investment that helps us with virtually everything we do, so we can bring more from ourselves, participate in activities more fully and live comfortably and healthily into old age.

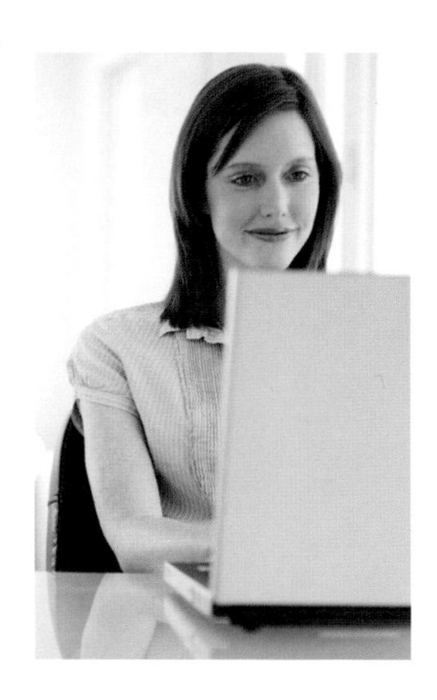

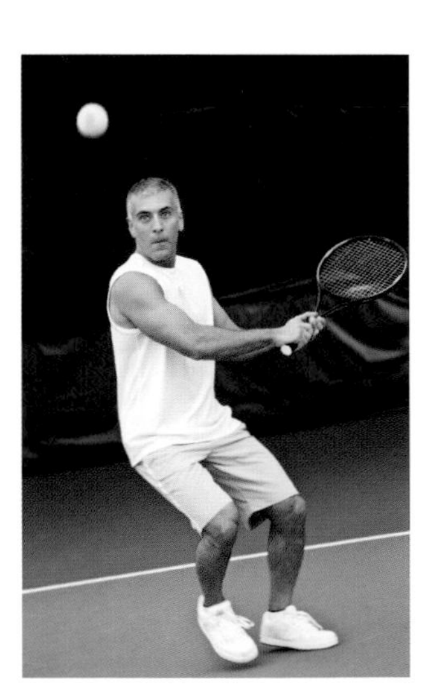

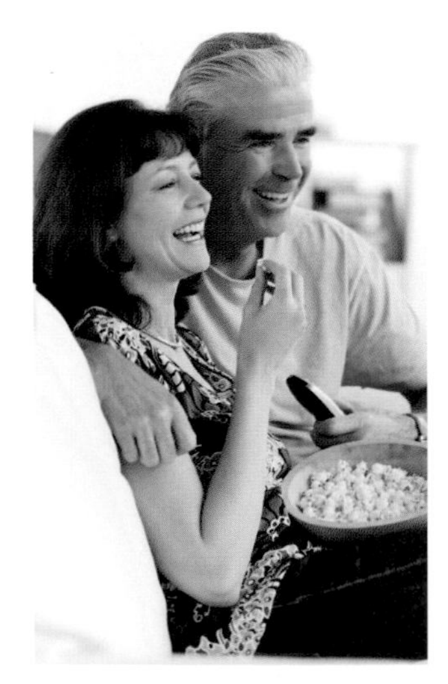

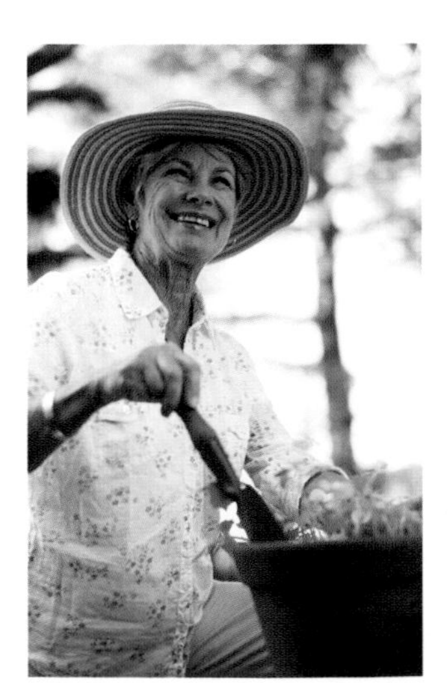

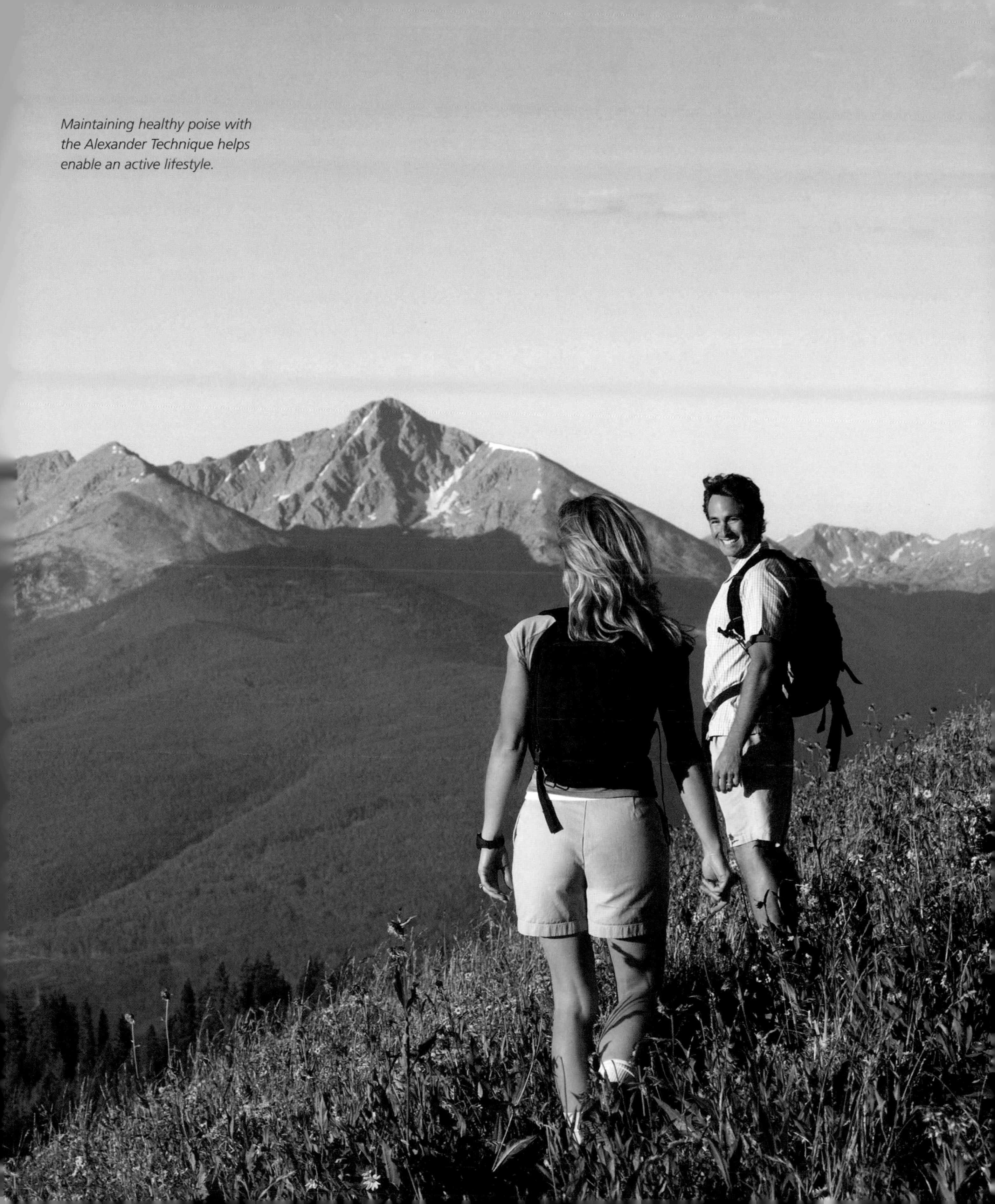

Maintaining healthy poise with the Alexander Technique helps enable an active lifestyle.

Improve your sport

Playing sport of any kind puts huge demands on us. Whether we run, swim, play tennis, golf, squash, football, rugby, cricket or badminton, we are pushing ourselves to achieve our best. Naturally we need to be fit for the task, so regular exercise is important for us to have the strength and stamina required, a healthy diet will support us and adequate sleep will refresh us. This is all in addition to the need to hone our skills in our game.

There is an important element to sporting ability that is often overlooked because it is not adequately recognised – the need for a well co-ordinated body. It may seem as if we are already adequately co-ordinated as we can walk in a straight line, thread a needle or hit the bull's eye in darts. But I would suggest that if you have postural habits that cause you to slouch or stiffen up and have back pain during your daily activities, you will also bring these same habits to your sport.

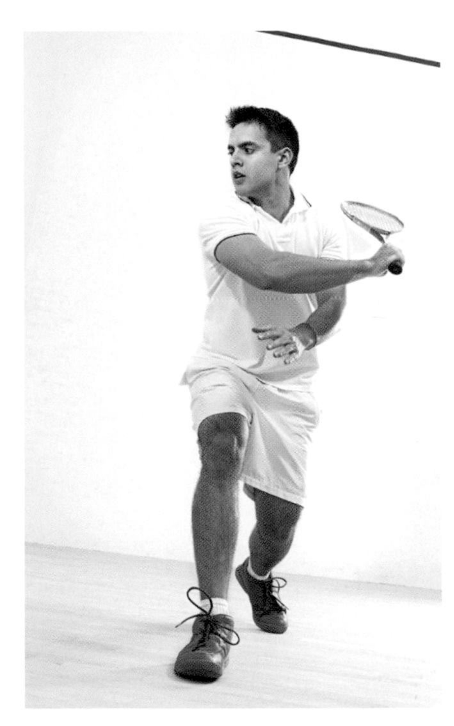

For instance, if you tend to lean forward or stoop a little when walking or running, you put yourself off balance and consequently your whole body is under strain. You will be stiffening your hips, calves and lower back just to prevent yourself from falling over. If you're a tennis player or golfer, you will swing your racquet or club with far more ease and with greater accuracy if you can do so without tensing your neck and shoulders unnecessarily.

The Alexander Technique helps free up our joints so we can move more easily, with greater speed and less wear and tear. We become more flexible throughout our torso so we can twist and turn more easily. We will run faster, get to the ball quicker and swing the club more accurately and fluidly. If we are at our full height and stature and free of habitual tension, we are less likely to harm our back, trap a nerve, or put back muscles into spasm. We may also find that learning sporting skills comes more easily as we are better co-ordinated.

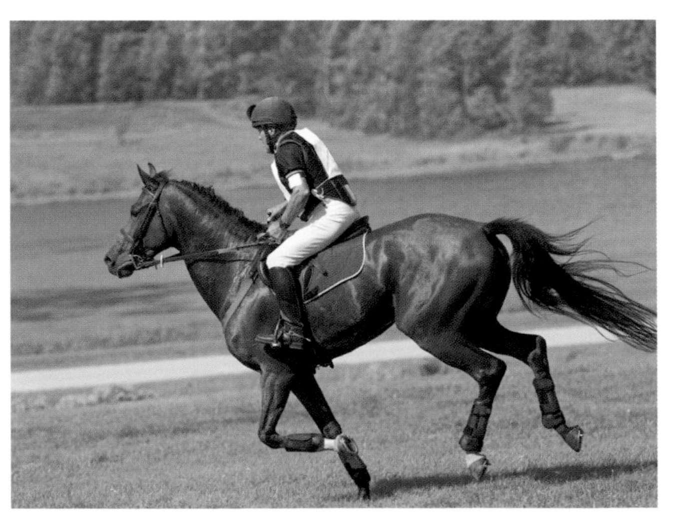

This brings to mind the need for a good coach and trainer who not only demonstrates high skill but also efficiency of movement and good poise too, as we learn by example.

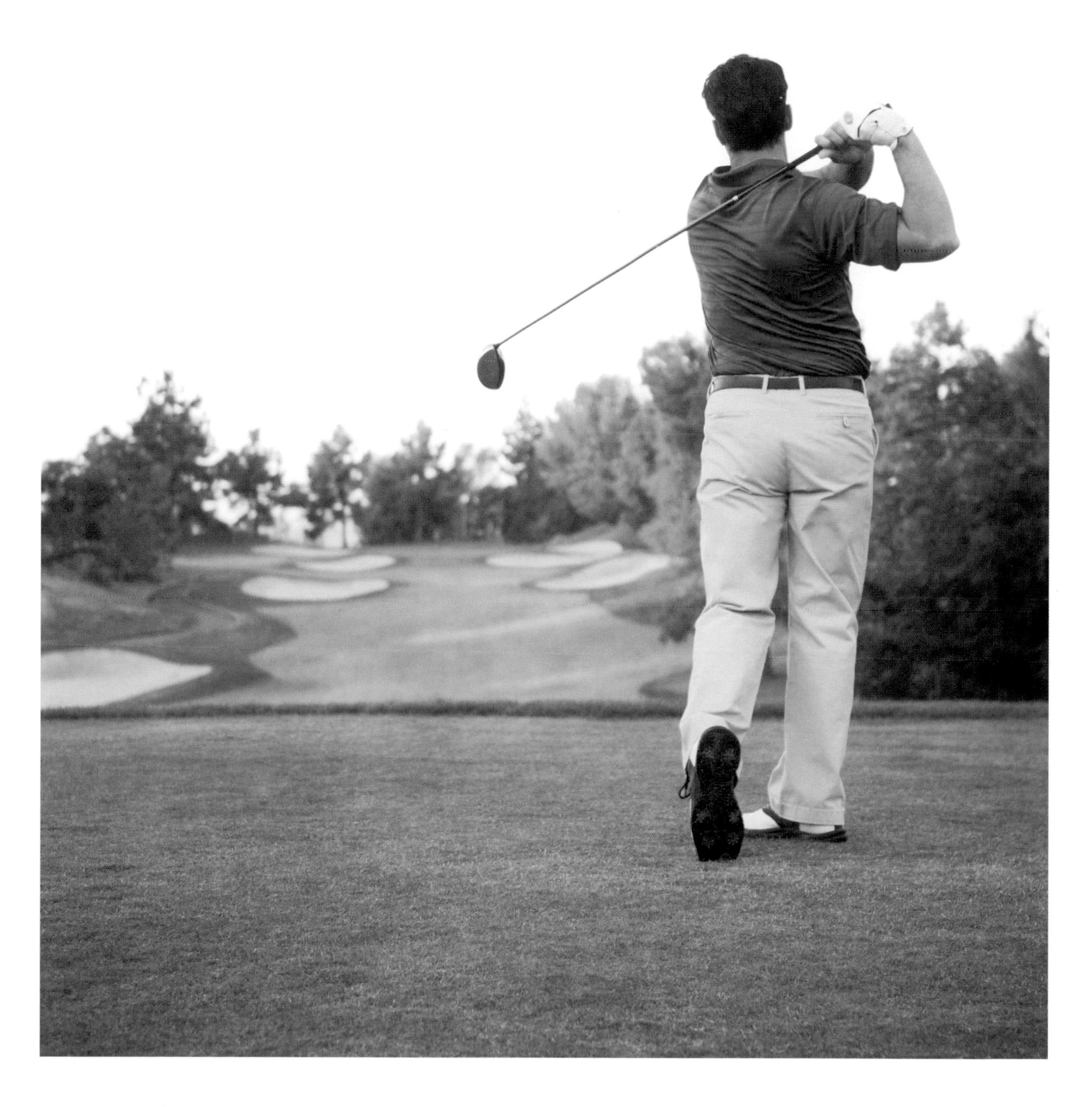

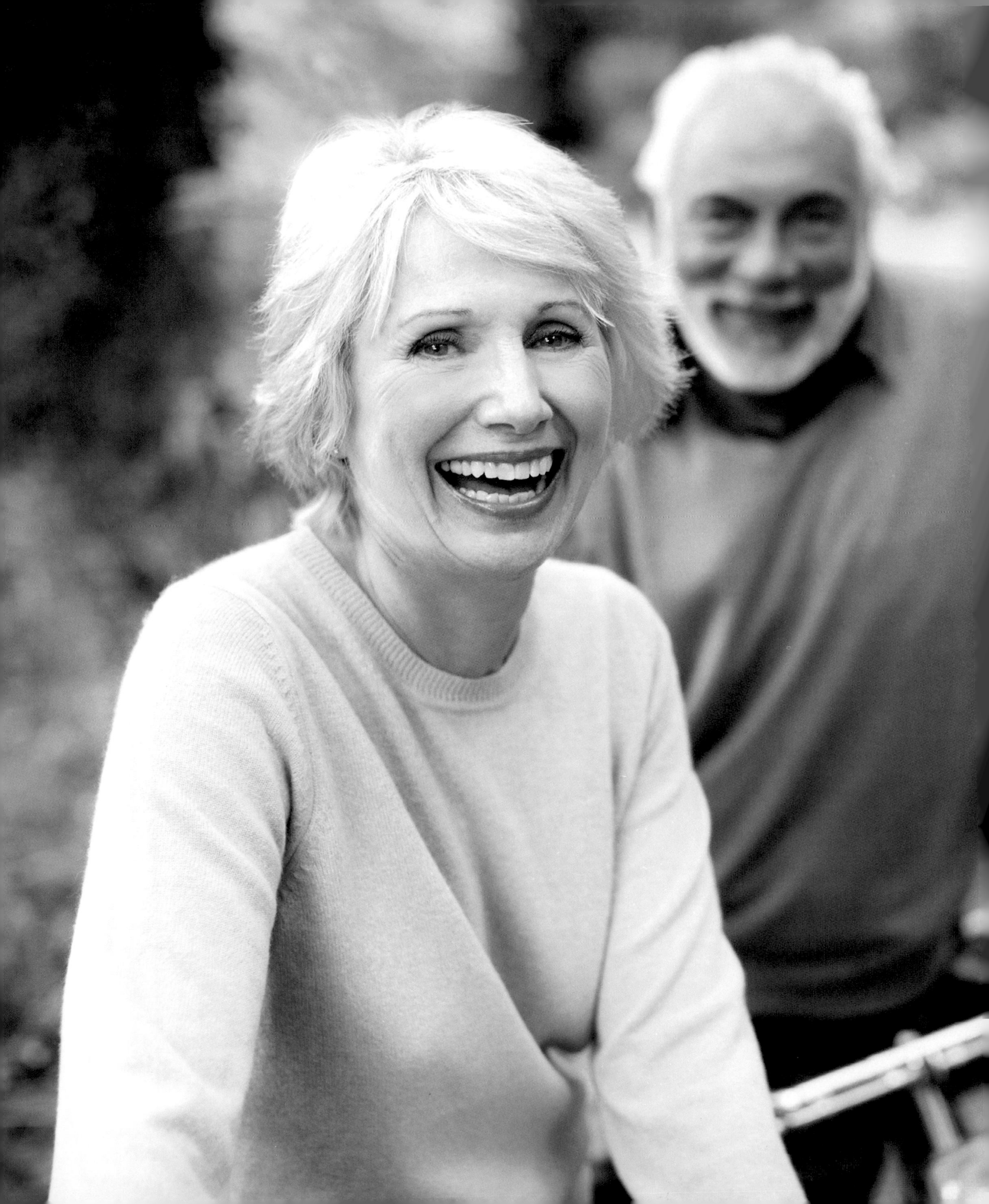

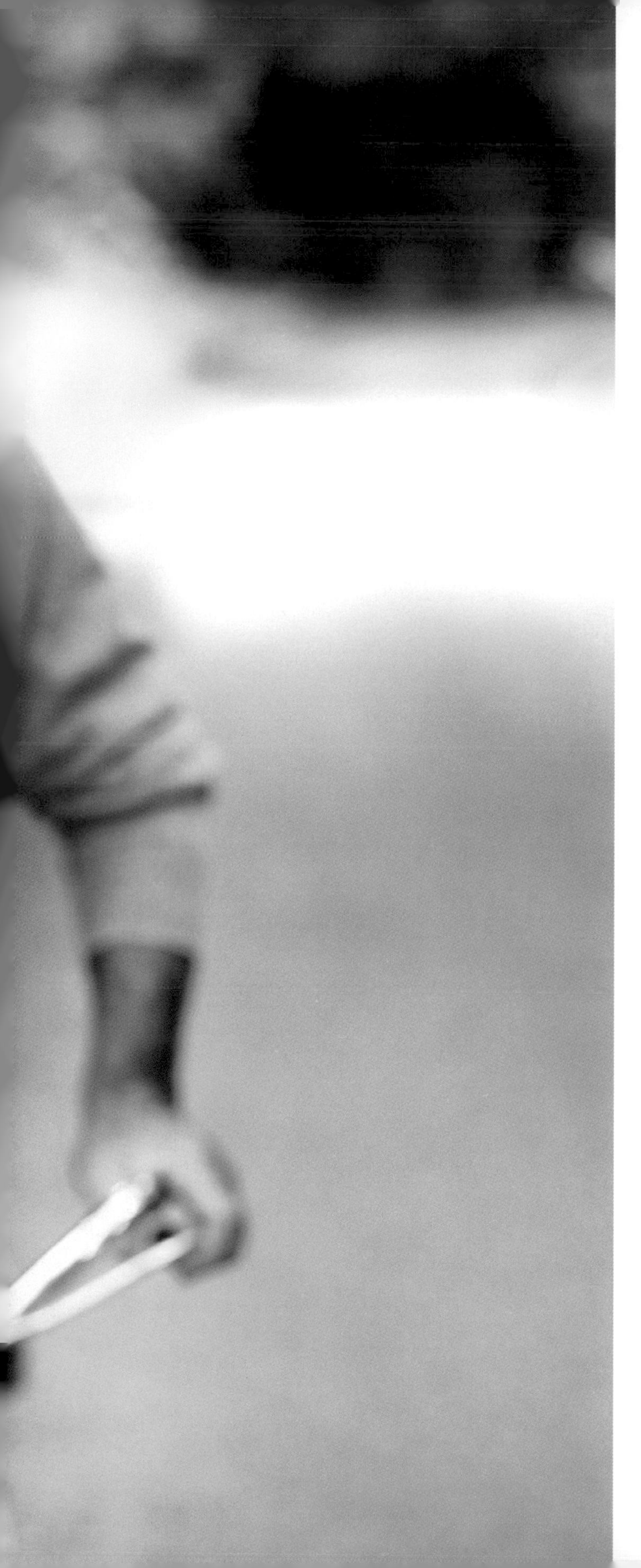

Look and feel younger

Having back pain of any sort can be wearing; we feel irritable and drained of energy. It reduces our mobility as we may stiffen to protect the area even without our awareness. The inability to carry heavy bags or even push the children's buggy makes us feel old beyond our years.

It's clear to see that if we're pain-free and able to move more easily and do all the domestic activities, as well as resume our favourite sport, we'll feel far fitter and more active. As we increase our activities and feel less protective of our injured or strained back it can feel like years have been lifted from us.

Learning and using the Alexander Technique helps restore youthful upright poise and makes us feel younger. It benefits our breathing by releasing unnecessary tensions which in turn helps to oxygenate the blood supply to aid healing and build collagen necessary for the elasticity of the connective tissue in our back. It also helps us eliminate toxins, clearing our skin so it's more translucent and less papery and our complexion a little more rosy. It also helps whiten our eyes, shine our hair and calm us down. We may even lose that worried frown!

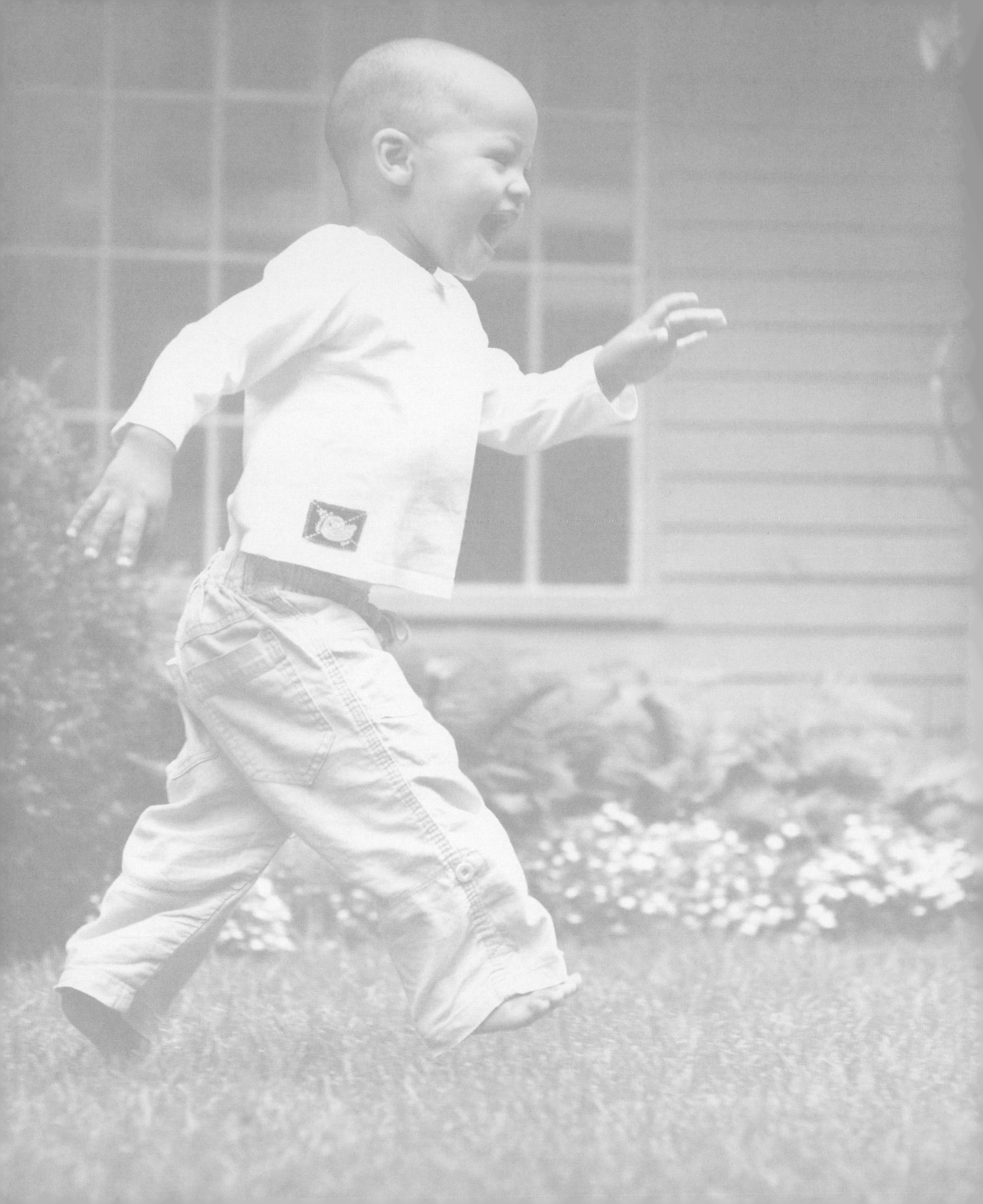

HABITS OF A LIFETIME

3

Developing bad habits

With time, we age and change in physique, health, stamina and strength. If we see our reflection in the mirror we may notice certain characteristics such as hunched shoulders, a possible tilt of the head to one side with one shoulder higher than the other, perhaps a slight twist, a hollowed or raised chest and slumped lower back. But were we always like this? If we retrieve some family photos from our early childhood, we'll probably see a healthy, happy and upright child who sits and stands tall and who is also very free and expansive. Unless we were disabled or injured, this is the way we all were, without postural habits as nature intended. Look at any young toddler and notice how upright and well poised they stand and sit and how freely they move around.

So, if we weren't born with postural habits when did they develop? We develop habits throughout our lifetime but they can even be observed in children as young as three or four. With repetition they become more ingrained so by the time we enter mid-life, we are just a more exaggerated version of how we were as a youngster. There are many influences on us that can affect our poise; we copy our parents irrespective of whether the examples we get are good or bad. If Mum shows us how to tie our shoe laces and she demonstrates by hunching her shoulders and stiffening her neck, then this is the example we copy; sitting in a twist at a school desk when writing and drawing will bring on scoliosis and slumping is the beginning of the cause of back pain. So, if we want to help our children avoid developing postural habits we should give them a good example!

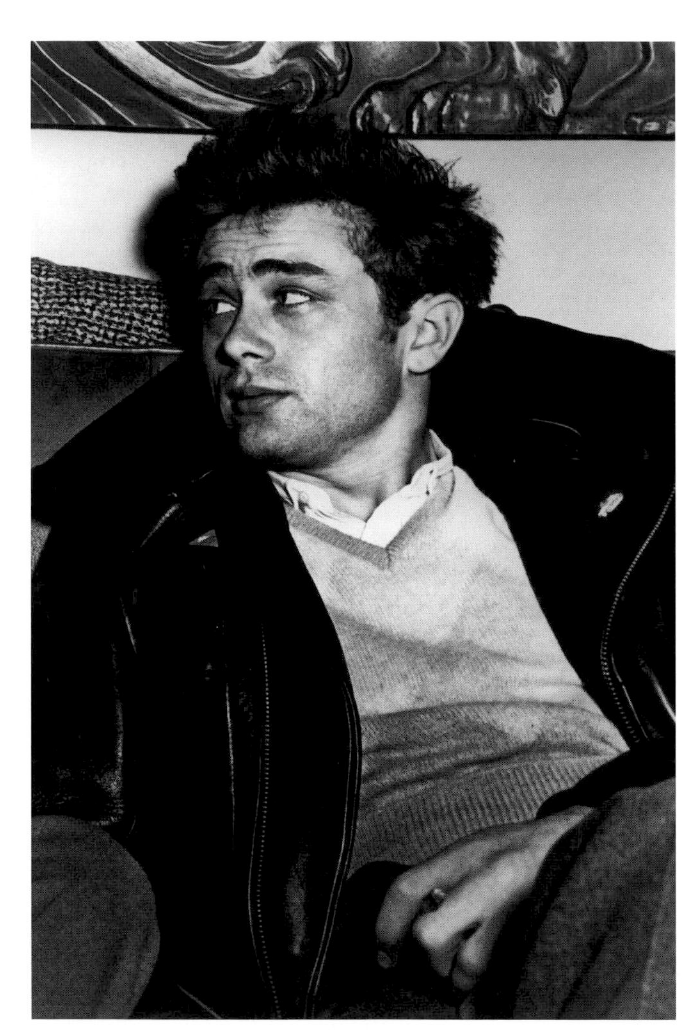

James Dean in typical cultured slouch.

Pubescence brings many emotional situations that can affect us: we may be unnervingly tall for our age so we stoop to hide our height, we may be self-conscious about other aspects of our appearance so we shrink into ourselves, or we may copy film stars, rock stars and our friends; it's thought to be 'cool' to hang out and slouch. James Dean has a lot to answer for in this respect having developed the 'cultured slouch'. Whatever manner we begin to hold ourselves in gets into our muscle memory and becomes an ingrained habit; the more we repeat it the more pronounced it becomes. With repetition we develop over-strong muscles in certain parts of our body, such as neck and upper back, purely because they have been overused, while others are underused.

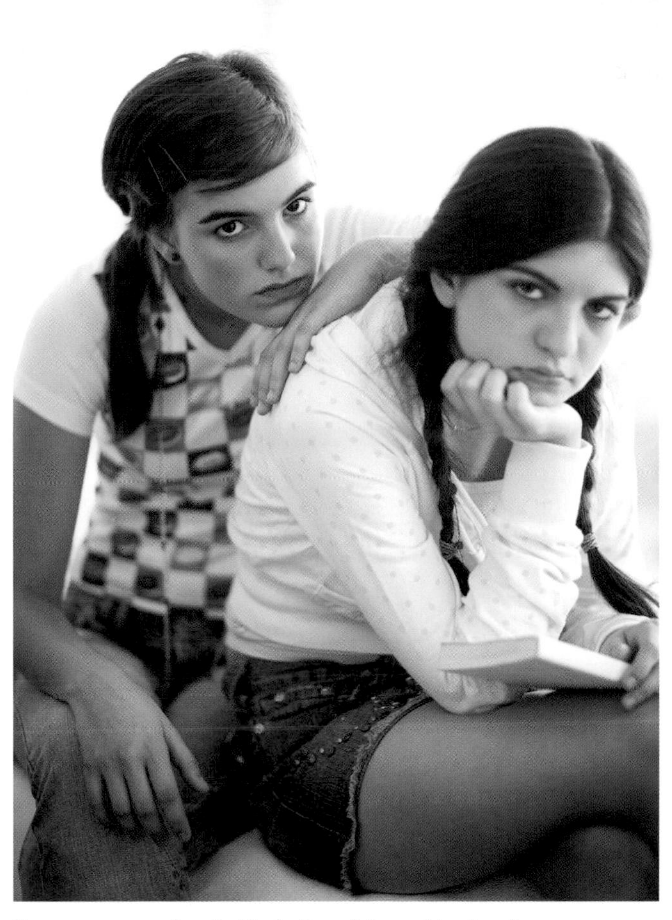

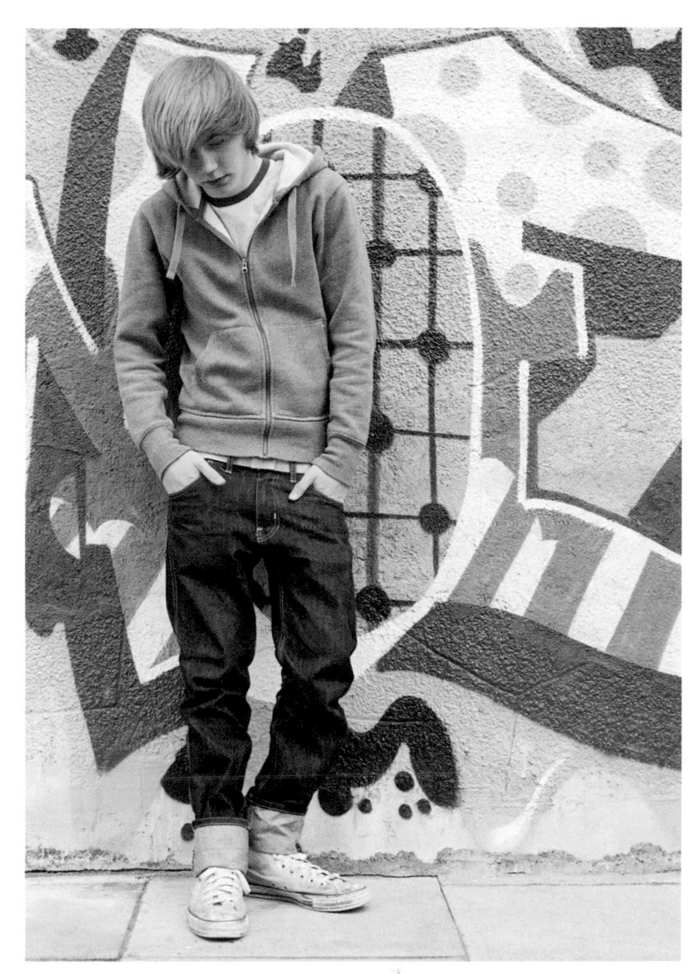

Teenagers are often led to believe it is cool to slouch, unaware or uncaring of the problems this will cause in the future.

No matter how old we are, however, we still have the instinct for healthy posture with which we were born. This instinct for poise is most clearly observed when a foal or calf is born and within minutes it attempts to stand up before it can even see clearly. It doesn't copy its mother; it needs to stand and walk very soon after birth to survive in the wild. We have a similar instinct for poise, and the extended time we allow our children to crawl on all fours in the first year or two helps the development of their hand, eye and brain co-ordination and their intelligence. I have given Alexander Technique lessons to people in their nineties and over who have become more upright, have restored their balance and who breathe more easily as we tap into this instinct – so it's never too late. It's about unlearning the old harmful habits we've picked up during our lifetime that interfere with our poise.

> We can throw away the habits of a lifetime in a few minutes if we use our brain. F.M. Alexander

It is sometimes said, 'You can't teach an old dog new tricks!' Well, my pupils demonstrate the contrary. We are not learning new 'tricks'; we are unlearning bad habits and re-learning the healthy poise we had before!

Another thing that we have in our favour is that no matter how old we are, we still have the same psycho-physical mechanism that we had as a youngster; we have the same muscles and same bones all in the same place. Our proportions may have changed, our legs may be longer and our head not so large in relation to our body size and our weight distribution will have altered too, but we are still standing on those two little feet that work all day to support us.

If we have the same instinct for healthy poise within us and the same skeletal musculature, then what has changed and why do we have an aching back? I would suggest it is the manner in which we use ourselves in daily life; how we use our musculature to move around, to support us as we sit or stand; how all of our hundreds of muscles co-ordinate together. Some muscles are doing far more than they should or need to do and others are not doing enough; we have an imbalance of effort going on and it is this that affects how we feel and function. For many of us, there is nothing wrong with our back per se despite possible pain, but there is something wrong with our muscular co-ordination. Top athletes, musicians and other performers all know the benefit of fine-tuning their muscle co-ordination as it can make the difference between a mediocre or a superb performance; the need for good co-ordination and balance shows itself clearly where expertise is important. And while we may not be 'performing' as such during our normal day, we are nevertheless still living with gravity. So unless we are in good balance and using our physique in healthy co-ordination, we will suffer the strains and effects on our health and well-being.

We tend to shorten our stature by stooping, contracting muscles and collapsing in the most harmful ways. We compress our hip joints, legs and throughout the length of our spine. Our shoulders may not rest in balance on the top of our ribcage as they should, putting pressure on our neck and upper back. Most of us contract our neck muscles virtually all the time, so our head is pulled backward off balance affecting our overall poise. All these tensions and habits undermine us so we can never bring the best of ourselves to our activities, never mind cope with the simple act of standing. When it comes to sitting, we are not physically well equipped for such an artificial position, yet we hope to survive hours a day for a whole working life, without giving our body any help or assistance to cope.

During the day, our muscles are working in support and movement; they are shortening and pulling one part of us toward another. This is all very well when we want to bend an arm or leg and we contract our flexor muscles, but we need to also allow other muscles – i.e. our extensor muscles – to release at the same time. Conversely when we intend to straighten a bent leg, or if we wish to stand upright, we need to release the contracted flexor muscles as we utilise the extensors to do the straightening. But if the opposing muscles are unable to adequately release for whatever reason, we will cause compression and excessive wear and tear to our joints. We will therefore be unable to come up to our full height and stature.

Slouching occurs when the back muscles give way and cease to support us while muscles in our front may be over-contracted, pulling us forward and down. We may be also narrowing our chest, hunching our shoulders and stiffening our neck. Slouching or stooping effectively reduces the internal capacity of our thorax so our internal organs have less space to function. On the other hand, if we try hard to hold ourselves up by bracing our back and pulling our shoulders back, we are again interfering with the very subtle muscular co-ordination that we rely on for healthy living; we will be using the wrong muscles to hold ourselves up and we become exhausted. Trying hard to maintain upright posture results in over-stiffening of muscles so they tire and we increase wear and tear. Sitting in a twist causes severe imbalance of the body and not only brings about back pain, but also sciatica, digestive problems and a hump on one side of the back.

It is my belief that one of the greatest causes of back pain – but also of many health problems to do with breathing, digestion, bowel and reproductive systems, depression and lethargy – is our tendency to shorten in stature by slumping or slouching forward. We shorten the vertical distance from our groin to our throat as we stoop downward by a combination of collapse of supportive muscles mostly in our back and excessive contractions of others around the chest and abdomen. The tendency may be caused partly by the lifestyle we lead, sitting at a desk for too many hours a day, leaning over the kitchen sink, slumping in front of the TV, cycling and even feeling depressed. Also, if we do a large number of 'sit-ups' and 'stomach crunches' without adequately stretching out afterwards, we can become severely compressed and shortened in our torso. Many of these tendencies set themselves up during our childhood as we copy our parents or friends and progressively get worse by repeated practice as the years go by. The phrase 'like father, like son' carries more than a grain of truth. Much of what we learn is from observing our parents, and mimicking; we pick up their tensional habits as we learn by example. Our body and mind do not distinguish between good example or bad; we learn it all!

By collapsing our back and constantly sitting in a slump, we lose the natural lumbar curve of our spine and can effectively reverse it so that it becomes convex rather than concave as nature intended. We can severely compress the discs so that they bulge and put pressure on a nerve and over time they can perforate so the disc ruptures. By stooping or slouching in such a way, we effectively put out of gear the supportive muscles that are intended to hold us upright all day, so they no longer function as they should, and other muscles have to come into play and do the best they can to prevent our unbalanced body from falling over. However, many of these muscles are not intended for long-term support as their main role is one of movement, so they soon become tired and stiff. We may now complain of backache.

Back pain is the tip of the iceberg. If we look beyond the pain, it is likely we will find that our posture and other aspects of our health are not as good as we might like. Poor posture also affects the healthy working of all our organs, resulting in problems with breathing, digestion, circulation, blood pressure, headaches, migraines, depression, irrational anger, lethargy, anxiety, timidity and low self-esteem. It will also impair our ability to perform as well as we might at sport, music, dance, public speaking, horse riding and virtually any activity that requires good co-ordination, balance and functioning.

There are more reasons why we develop postural habits and one very major one is that we do not take care not to fall into bad habits because we have no awareness of it happening!

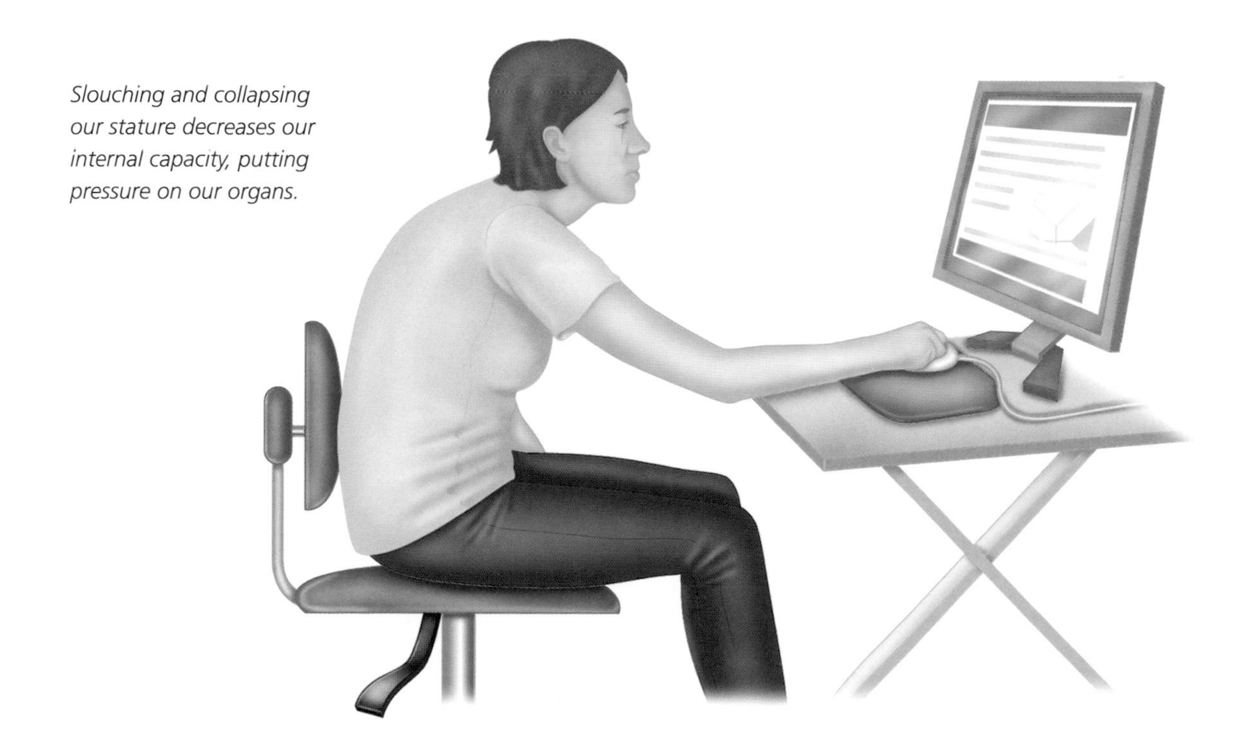

Slouching and collapsing our stature decreases our internal capacity, putting pressure on our organs.

Observe yourself

When it comes to posture, we don't give it much thought except when we perhaps try on a new suit or when it lets us down and we get backache. F.M. Alexander discovered when he started investigating his own vocal problems that he was using himself incorrectly.

He first deduced that he was doing something wrong when he spoke, and that view was endorsed by doctors and voice specialists, but they were unable to advise him as to exactly what the problem was, so he decided to find out for himself. He set up a mirror so he could see what he was doing when he spoke, and eventually he placed a further two mirrors so he could see different angled reflections of himself, from the side and behind. We may not have three large mirrors to hand, but if we have one, we could use that in a similar way to Alexander to see our own situation.

> All the darned fools in the world believe they are actually doing what they think they are doing. F.M. Alexander

The hardest thing about using a mirror in the manner that Alexander did is resisting being distracted by the state of our hair, our expanding waistline, or any other physical characteristic we may feel is undesirable. So when you look in the mirror, don't suck your stomach in and pull your shoulders back or do anything at all; just observe. Look and see what you can see, dispassionately, objectively and without being critical. Doing this alone is quite a challenge. In the Alexander Technique lesson, the teacher provides hands-on guidance so we begin to notice what we are doing.

It is good to notice every aspect of our poise, as we sit, stand and walk. By observing we notice our habits and what we are doing to ourselves. Alexander's habit when he spoke was to pull his head backward, depress his larynx and stiffen his neck. Later he discovered that he needed to inhibit these harmful tendencies before he could then bring about a better use of himself.

Before you continue and discover how to use the Alexander Technique in detail, ask yourself: 'How am I using myself right now?' Wherever you are, sitting at your desk, in a chair at home, or standing in a queue at a checkout, pay attention to yourself and notice what you are doing. Try to observe what it is that you are doing as you sit or stand, without actively doing something about it. Just observe.

Line yourself up with the edge of a mirror and observe if you are upright or leaning.

HELPFUL TIP

›› Any adjustment you may make to your posture, such as pulling yourself up straight, will not improve your co-ordination or restore your natural poise. You are simply pulling yourself around. Try to dispassionately observe how you are. Look in a mirror and notice any posture tendency you have. If you can do this without reacting, you are already beginning to use 'Inhibition', the cornerstone of the Alexander Technique.

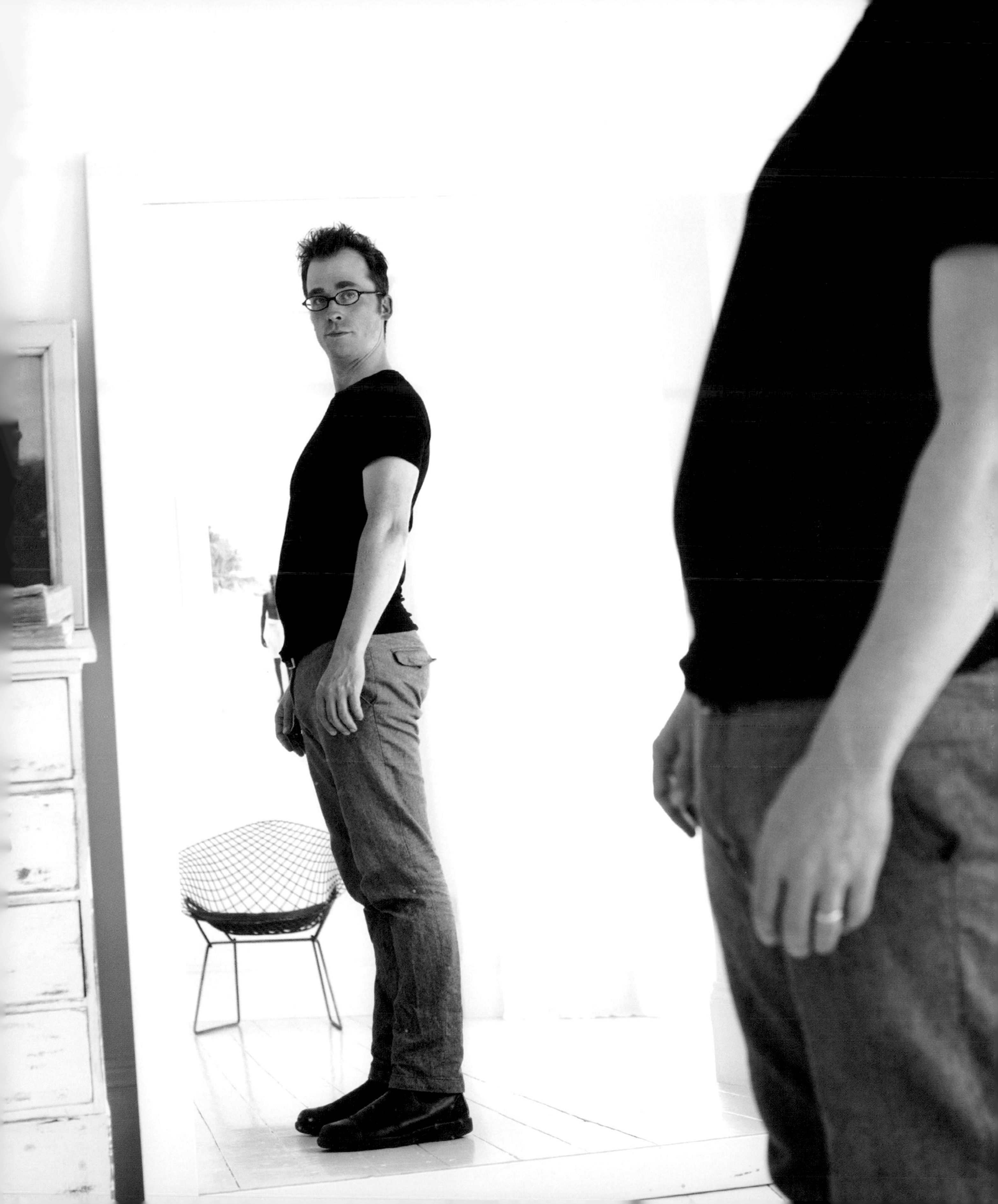

Exercise

›› Observe how you are sitting or standing without making any adjustments. 'Inhibit' adjusting yourself to look or feel correct. See if you can notice any postural habits you might have such as sitting in a twist. Are your shoulders raised or one higher than the other, are you collapsed in a slouch, are you dropping your head and neck forward and pulling your head backward? Are you pushing your hips forward when standing and arching your back, or are you standing rather stiffly and held in an attempt to be upright? Are you sitting with your legs wrapped around the leg of the chair, or are you sitting on your legs folded underneath you, which may reduce good circulation?

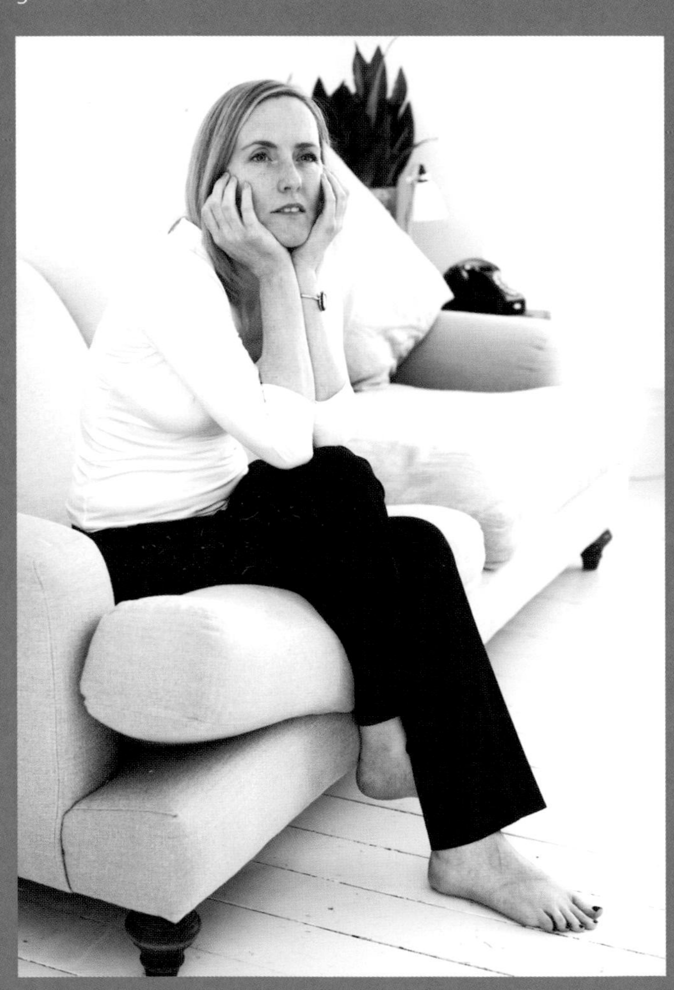

Sitting slumped with rounded shoulders and legs twisted.

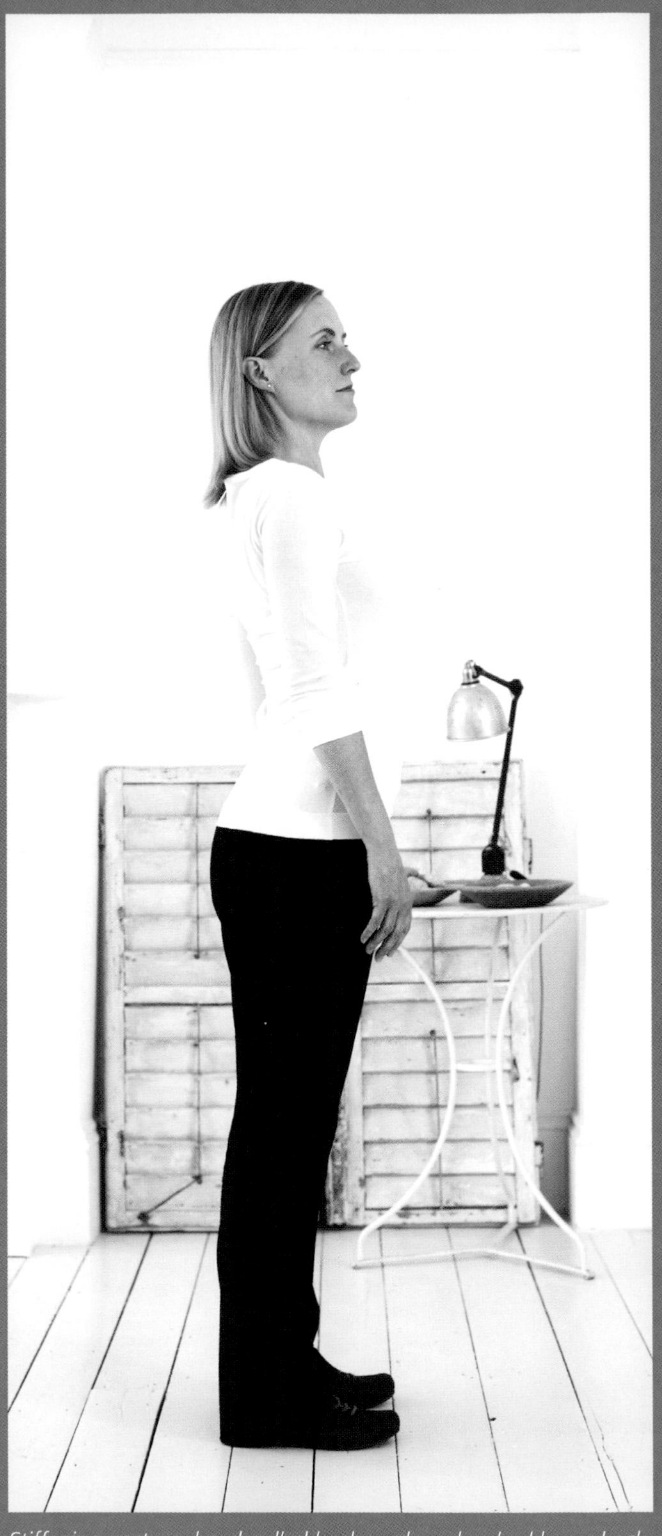

Stiffening posture, head pulled backwards and arched lower back.

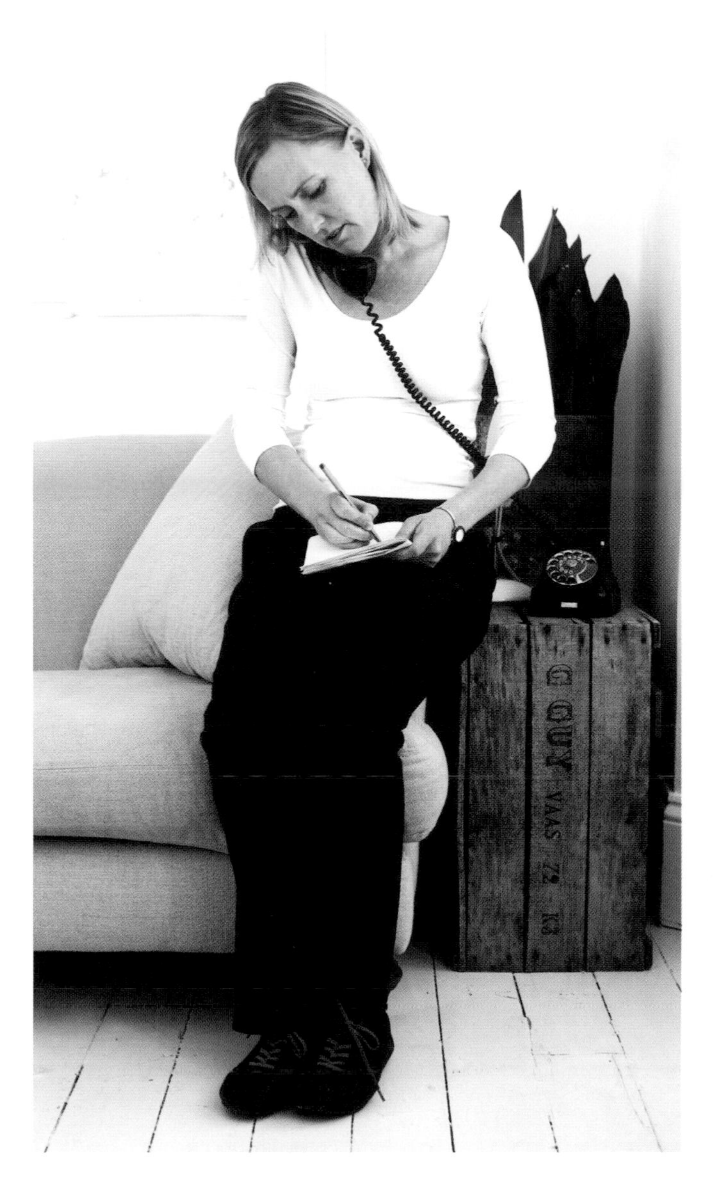

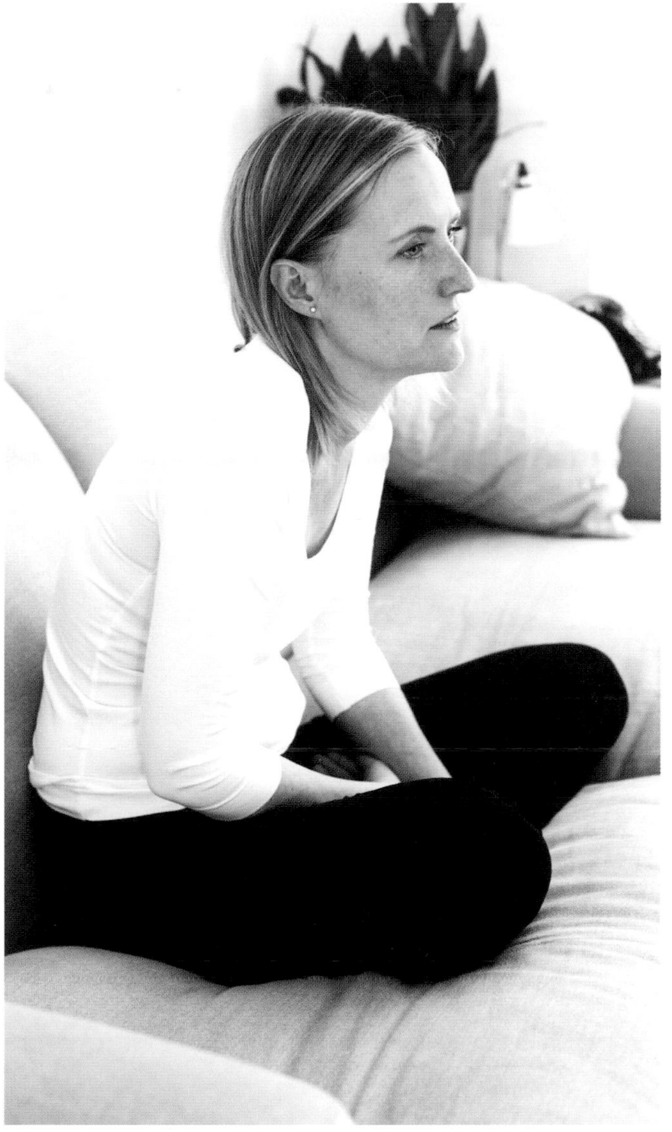

l. *One shoulder raised, neck twisted and collapsed stature.*
r. *Slumped back, stiff neck and head pulled back, sitting on legs.*

Being aware of our posture is half the battle. There may be something simple we can do to help ourselves instantly without reading further on in this book. If you discover something obvious such as your shoulders raised up around your ears, then see if you can just release them so they drop; don't pull them down, but release the tension that is raising them. If your ankles are wrapped around the legs of the chair, unfurl them and let your feet rest flat on the floor in front of you. If you are standing unevenly with the weight of your body going down one leg rather than two, see if you can centre your weight so that you are even on both legs.

Balance

As soon as we start to consider our posture we come face-to-face with our balance and the Earth's gravitational pull. Gravity is working away the whole time, and we know without thinking too much about it that anything that is not in good balance will fall over. If we get a pile of bricks and stand them one on top of another to make a vertical column, we will soon discover that unless the stack is absolutely straight, the pile will eventually topple. The more irregular we make this column, i.e. by staggering the bricks to the left or right, and the higher it gets, the more likely it is to tumble.

If we stop for just a second, stand up and look down at our feet we will see that they are relatively small in relation to our overall height. Clearly if we do not stand in good balance we will either fall over or need to stiffen in some way to prevent ourselves from falling. As it happens, most of us are slightly off balance all the time and consequently stiffening to compensate; it is no wonder we end up with a painful backs.

If we look at the weight distribution of our body, we can see very quickly that our centre of gravity is high: for men it is in the lower chest and for women through the abdomen. In addition to all this our head weighs approximately 4–5kg (9–11lb), and to make matters worse our feet are small in relation to our height. We are top heavy so good balance is essential. Standing or sitting off balance can become such an ingrained habit that we do not know we are doing it. In order to avoid back pain and to make the most of ourselves in any situation – be it working in the office, playing sport or even just walking or bending – it is essential that we are in good balance, thus avoiding unnecessary strain. If we can become more aware of how we stand and sit, we can begin to change our habits.

If we stand upright so our weight is evenly distributed, shoulders over hips, over ankles, we are standing in better balance which will help us avoid back strain.

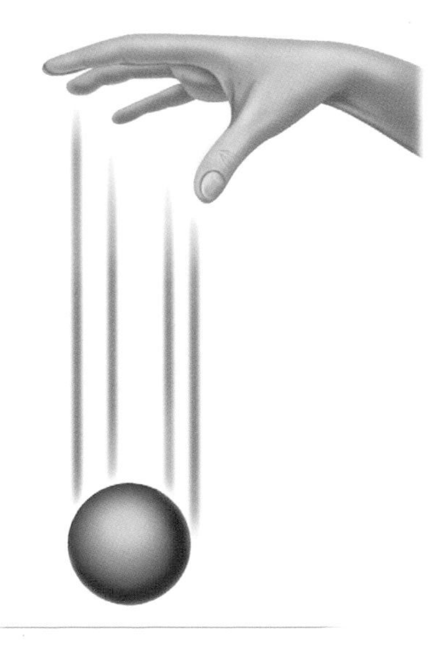

The Earth's gravitational pull is vertical.

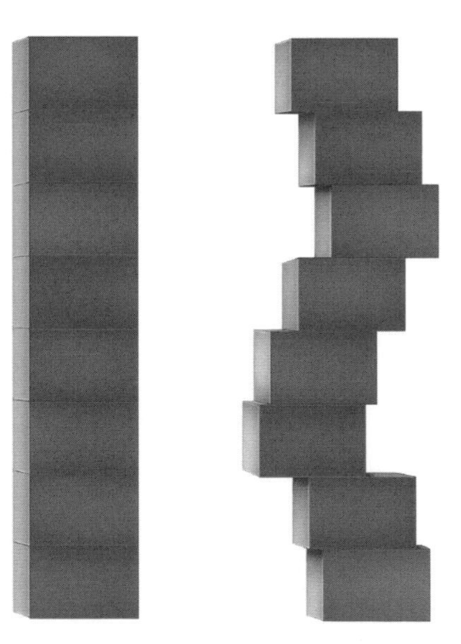

A pile of bricks built evenly and vertically is far more stable than an uneven pile which is under threat of toppling over.

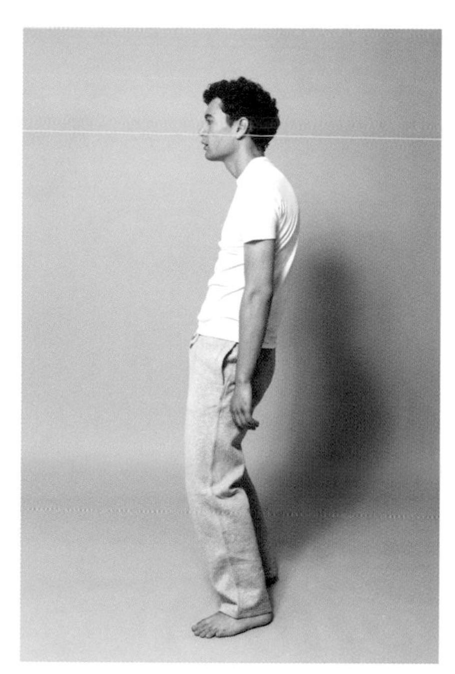

If we stand with our hips pushed forward, arching our back and hunching, we are off balance and under threat of falling. This causes huge strain to our back and neck.

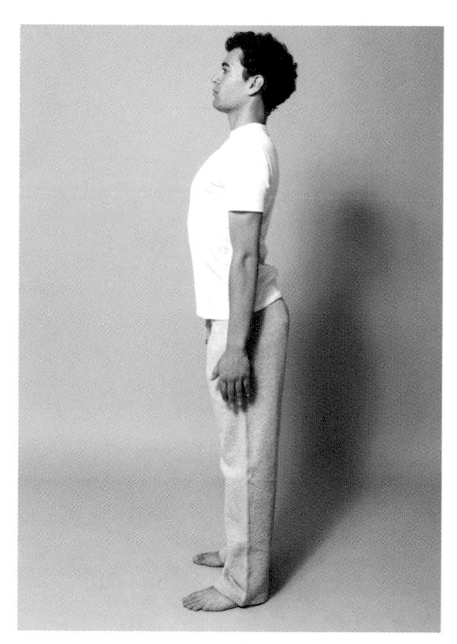

Trying hard to hold ourselves up causes unnecessary strain and stiffness, and is just as harmful as slouching.

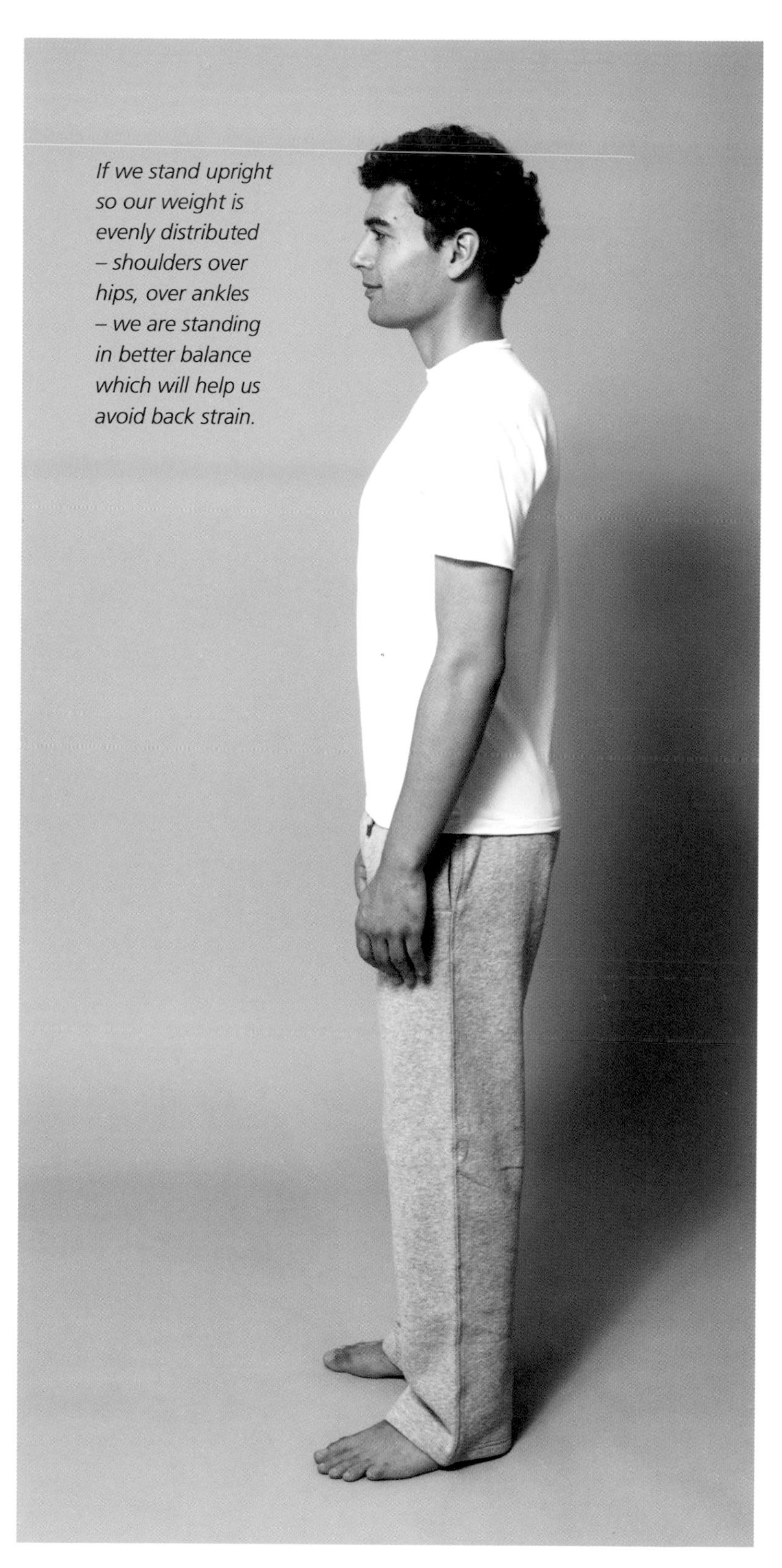

If we stand upright so our weight is evenly distributed – shoulders over hips, over ankles – we are standing in better balance which will help us avoid back strain.

Exercise – Faulty sensory perception

›› Stand with your weight evenly on both feet side-on in front of a mirror so you can see yourself in profile. Are you standing vertically or are you leaning forward or arching your back? Imagine you are the pendulum of a clock and allow yourself to sway forward and backward very slightly. Gradually reduce your sway until you feel that you are in balance standing vertically. Now look in the mirror to one side and just check if your senses are accurate (see page 43). Are you upright or are you still leaning? If you are still leaning, bring your body into vertical alignment by observing what you are doing in the mirror. Does it feel right? Now you are possibly more upright, see if you can relax some of the effort so you make less effort when standing than before.

›› Turn face-on to the mirror and ignore your hair, facial expression or any other distraction and notice, without doing anything, if your head is actually vertical or is it tilted to one side? Line up the side of your face with the edge of the mirror. See if you can centre your head so that it is straight. Does it feel straight or does this feel wrong?

›› Is one shoulder higher than the other? Let a raised shoulder drop down a little so they are more even. Does this feel wrong? Of course you may have one shoulder dropped too low but do not try to raise it as you will cause unnecessary tensions.

›› It's interesting how strange it feels if we change how we are holding ourselves when standing from our habitual stance to one that is not habitual but nevertheless more upright. This shows that we cannot trust our feelings, as our sensory perception has become faulty by repeating poor habits throughout our lives. However, as we refine our poise with the Alexander Technique our senses become more accurate.

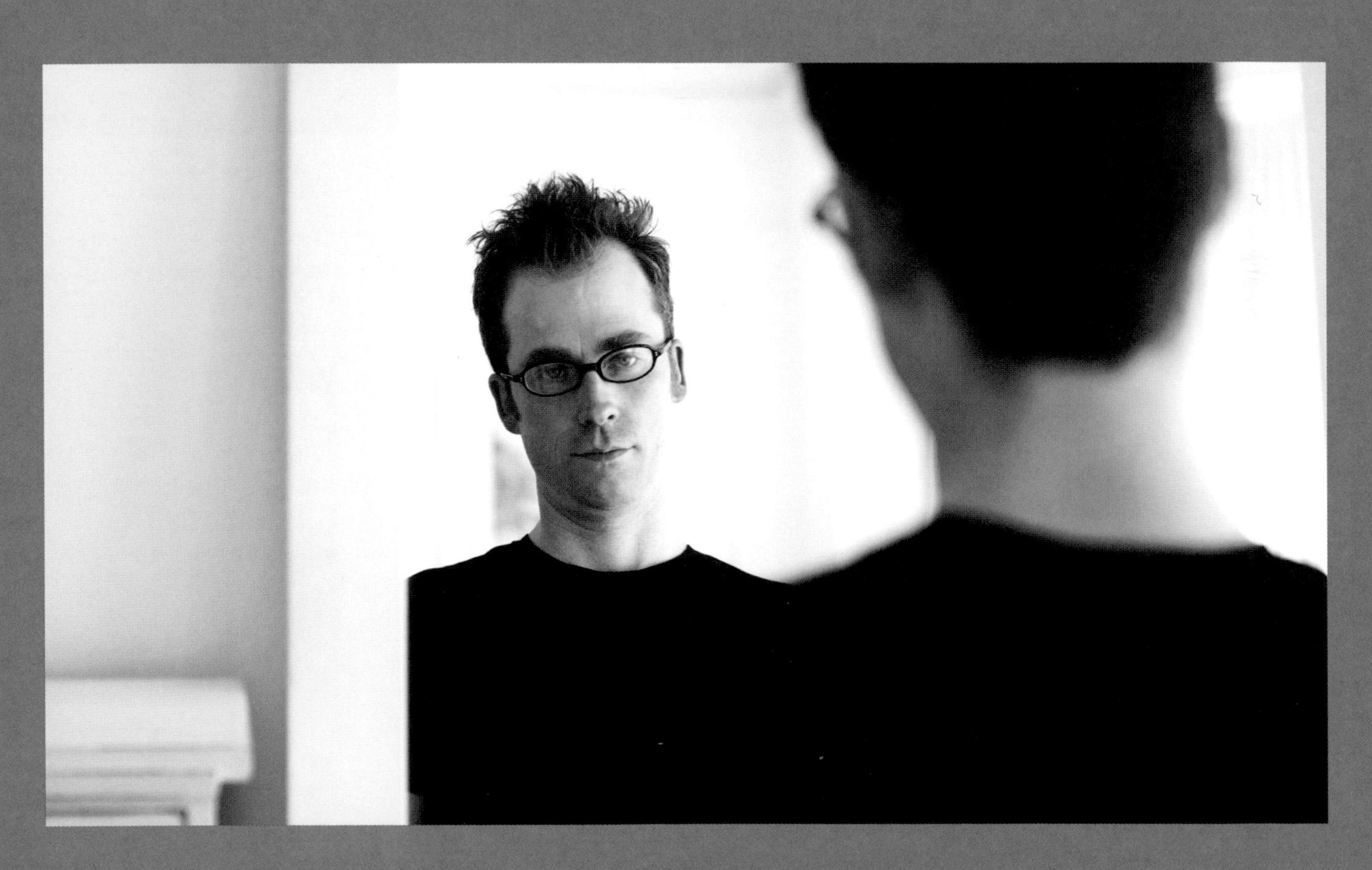

Developing an awareness of good balance

Maintaining good balance involves the effective working of the vestibular mechanism of the inner ear, our eyes to help our awareness of our position and the freedom of our neck. If you experience dizzy spells, you should visit a doctor so your inner ear can be examined. However the efficient working of the sub-occipital muscles under our skull requires our neck to be as free as possible, so that these small and sensitive muscles can give feedback to the cerebellum in our brain about our position in space.

We can help ourselves enormously by freeing our neck (discussed further in Chapter 4) as it will help improve not just the balance of our head but the balance of our entire body. Gradually the tendency to tighten our neck muscles becomes less with time and our awareness of balance and proprioception (our overall body sense) will be generally improved.

HELPFUL TIPS

›› An awareness of how your spine supports you can help you release unnecessary tension in your back.

›› If we look at the lumbar curve of our lower back, we can see that the vertebrae are very deep. The 'nobbles' you can feel along your spine are only the tips of the Transverse Process of each vertebra where muscles and ligaments attach. The weight bearing and supportive part of our lumbar spine is very close to the centre of the torso, but it is common to mistakenly believe that our spine is in our back (see illustration).

›› Just as an apple has a core through its centre, think of your spine passing through the middle of your torso as a central core. Think of your body 'surrounding' your spine so your torso is supported through the middle. Perceiving your torso to be supported in this way will help you release unnecessary tensions in your back.

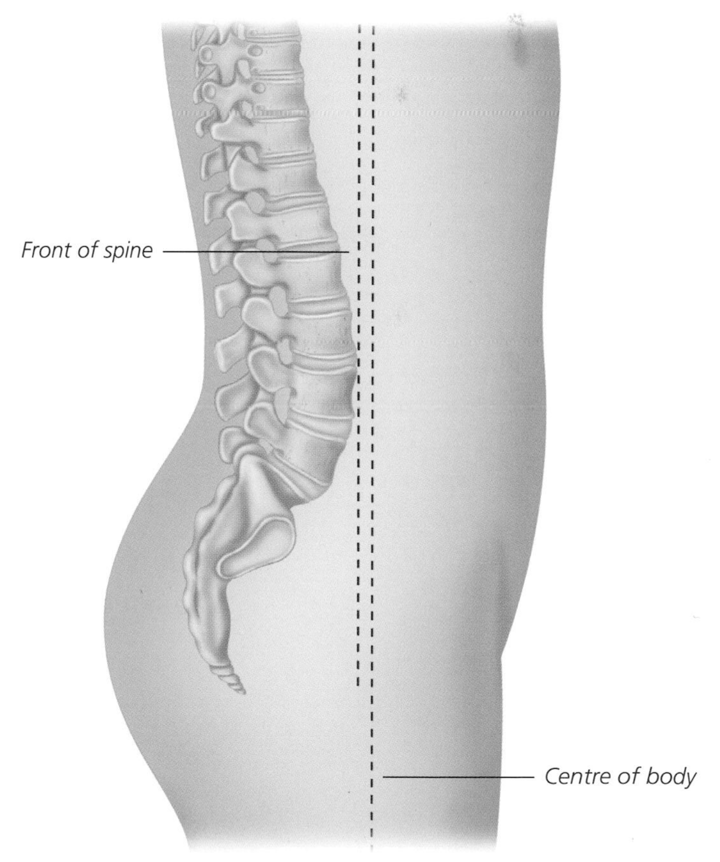

The front of the spine is very close to the centre of the body.

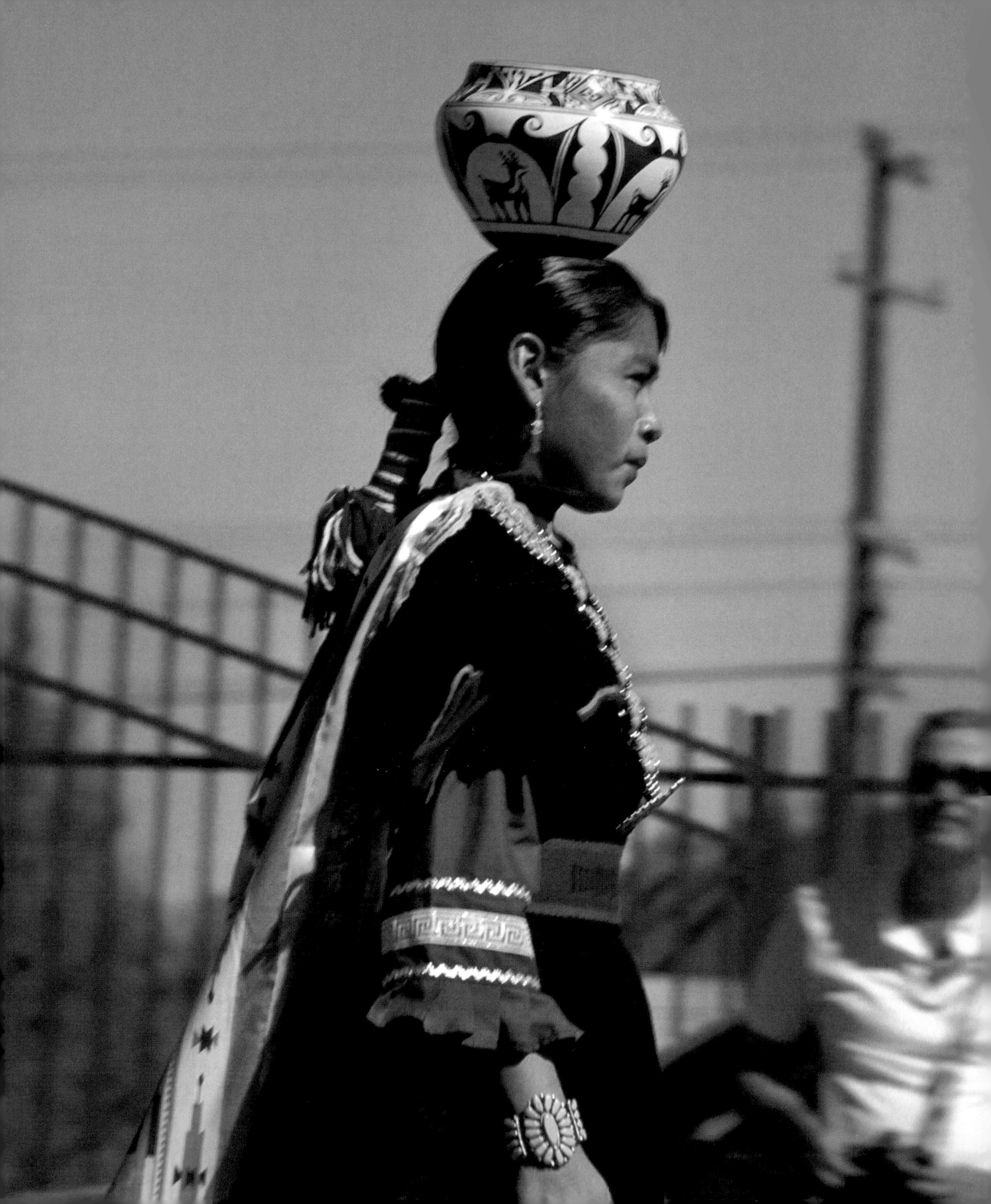

Good poise

In our developed society it is rare to come across someone with great natural posture as most of us pick up bad postural habits along the way. However sometimes we can be lucky enough to come across someone with inspiring natural poise.

Nuba tribespeople in southern Sudan also show great natural poise, as can be seen in the celebrated photograph below by George Roger, 1949. This heroic titan had just won a wrestling match and is seen riding on the shoulders of another young warrior. See how upright and broad he is, but his right hand and wrist show how free he is too.

In countries where people carry pots on their heads, we see wonderful examples of natural upright poise, which is necessary in order to bear such loads for any distance without strain.

So what is good poise? Given the evolution of the human species, good poise is a consequence of efficient use of our mechanism. It is when we are in good balance and can move with minimal effort while also retaining our fullest expansive stature for healthy internal functioning and movement. When these conditions exist, back pain will not occur. When we enjoy such a balanced and free expansive poise, we can truly bring the best from ourselves to any activity or performance. So, good poise is not about holding ourselves stiffly 'upright'.

This free expansive quality is desirable whether we are still, or walking, bending, twisting, dancing, running or doing any activity whatsoever. Good poise involves being in good balance while in movement. We can only have good balance if our joints are free and supple as this allows our body to easily adapt to changing circumstances during movement.

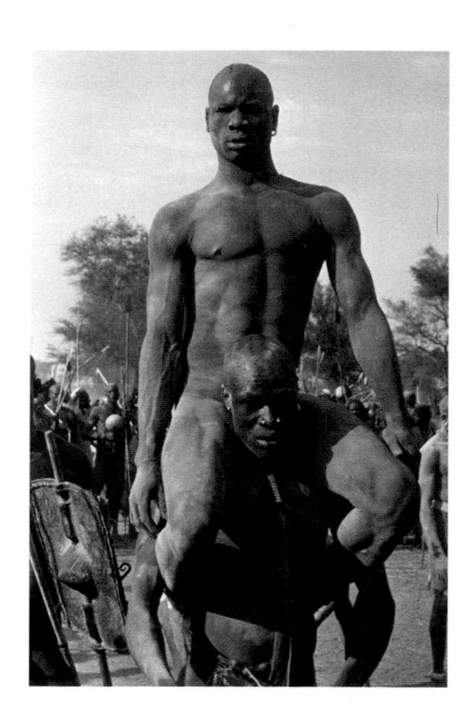

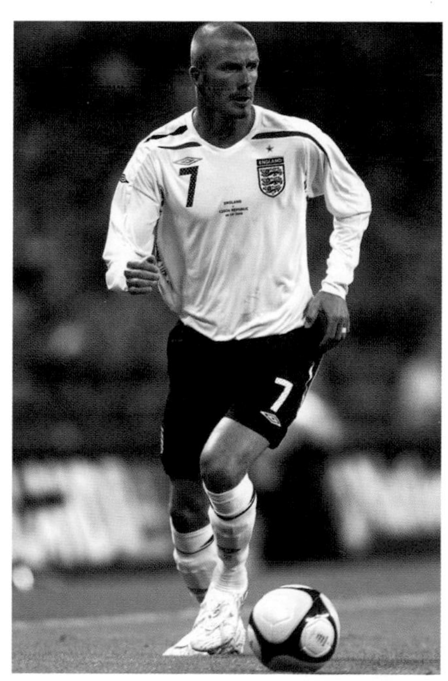

Wrestlers of the korongo Nuba tribe of Kordofan Sudan.

David Beckham demonstrates good co-ordination and poise.

Children have great poise

If we observe children between two and four years of age we will see examples of wonderful healthy upright posture. They stand tall at their full height; they bend easily at their knees and hips to squat; they run and twist and turn with grace and ease. How wonderful it would be to have that poise now. It's the way we are meant to be. Sadly from the age of four or five we develop postural habits such as stiffening our neck, collapsing our lumbar back as we slouch in chairs, we hunch our shoulders and do all manner of tensions as well as disengaging muscles that should support us.

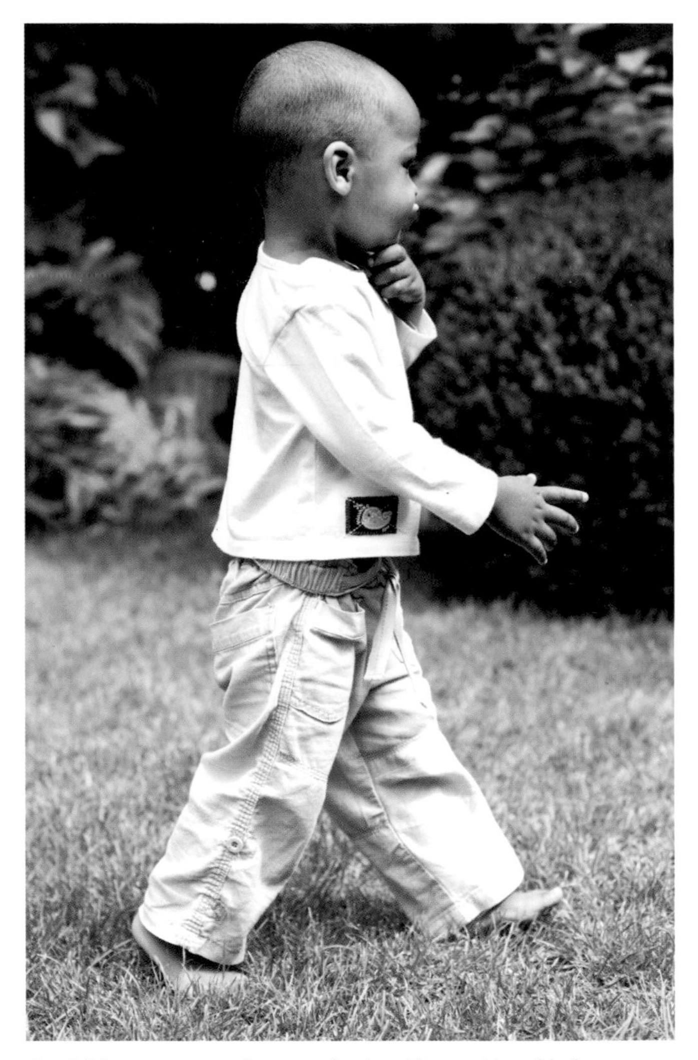

As children we naturally move freely with good head balance, and lengthen in stature as we walk.

But if we look at our physique today and compare it to how we were as very young children, we can see that there is not a great deal of difference. Although our size and proportions have changed, we still balance on two feet and we have the same musculature. If we had great poise then but not so now, what has changed is not our physique but the manner in which we use ourselves.

It is clear by looking at children that good posture is not contrived but something that happens naturally when we are free of bad postural habits that interfere with our subtle co-ordination. Back pain is nearly always an indication of loss of natural poise and the development of postural habits. We need to 'unlearn' our bad habits.

> Prevent the things you have been doing and you're half way home. F.M. Alexander

The process of consciously preventing poor postural habits from affecting us is a major aspect of the Alexander Technique and is referred to as 'Inhibition'. We will be discussing this at length in the next chapter.

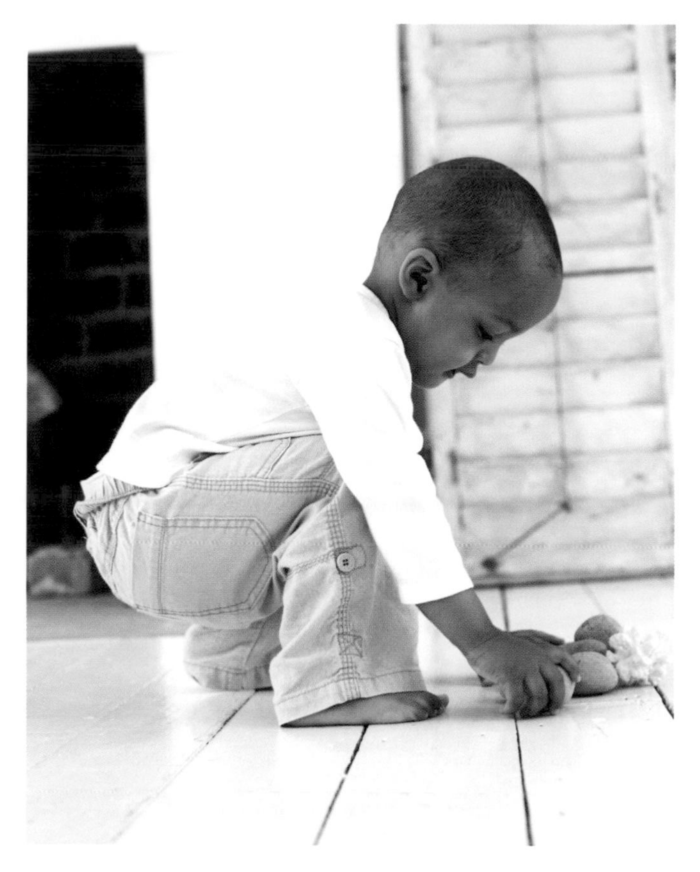

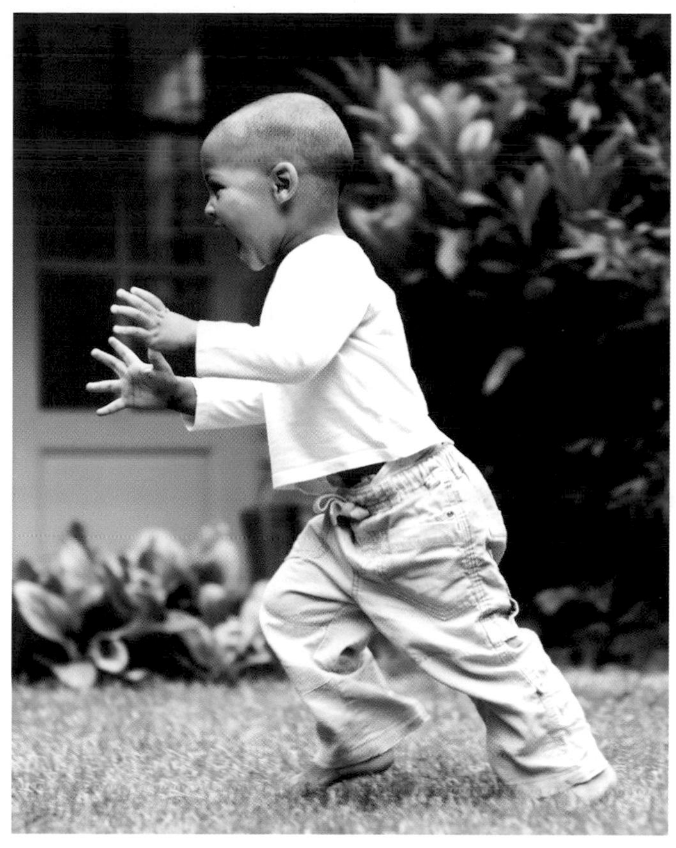

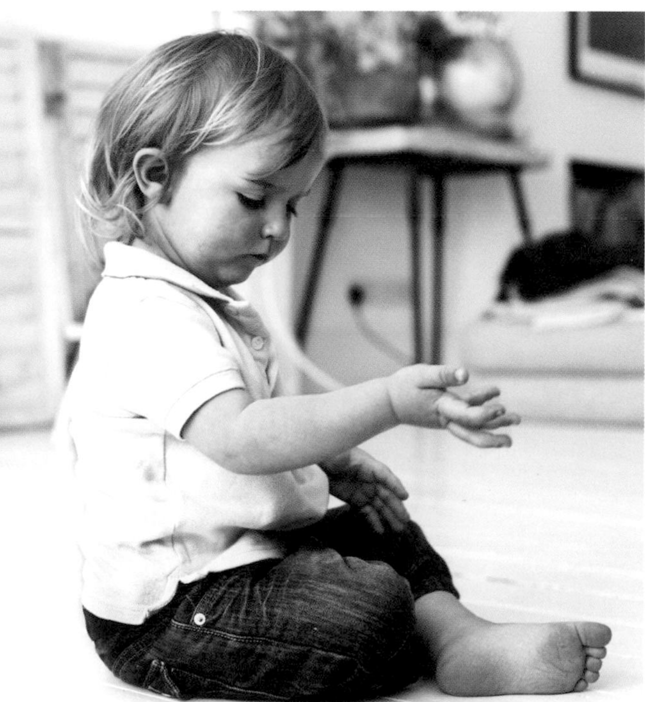

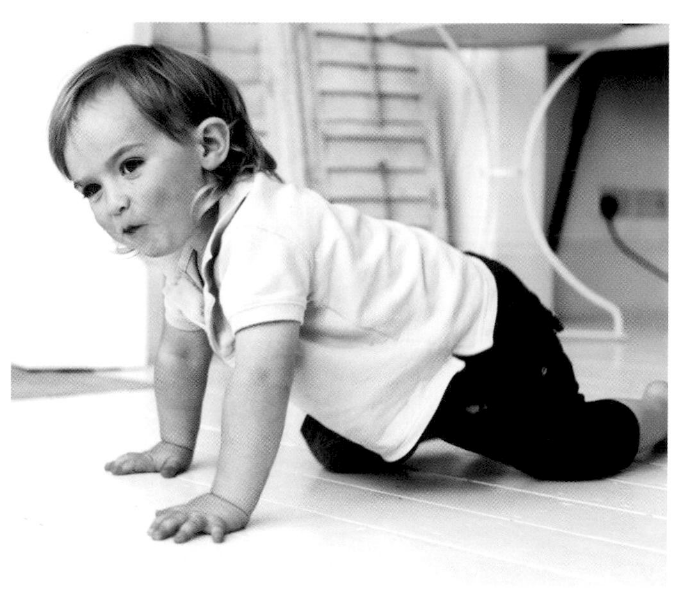

The Alexander Technique helps us to un-learn our bad postural habits so we can regain much of the natural poise we had as young children.

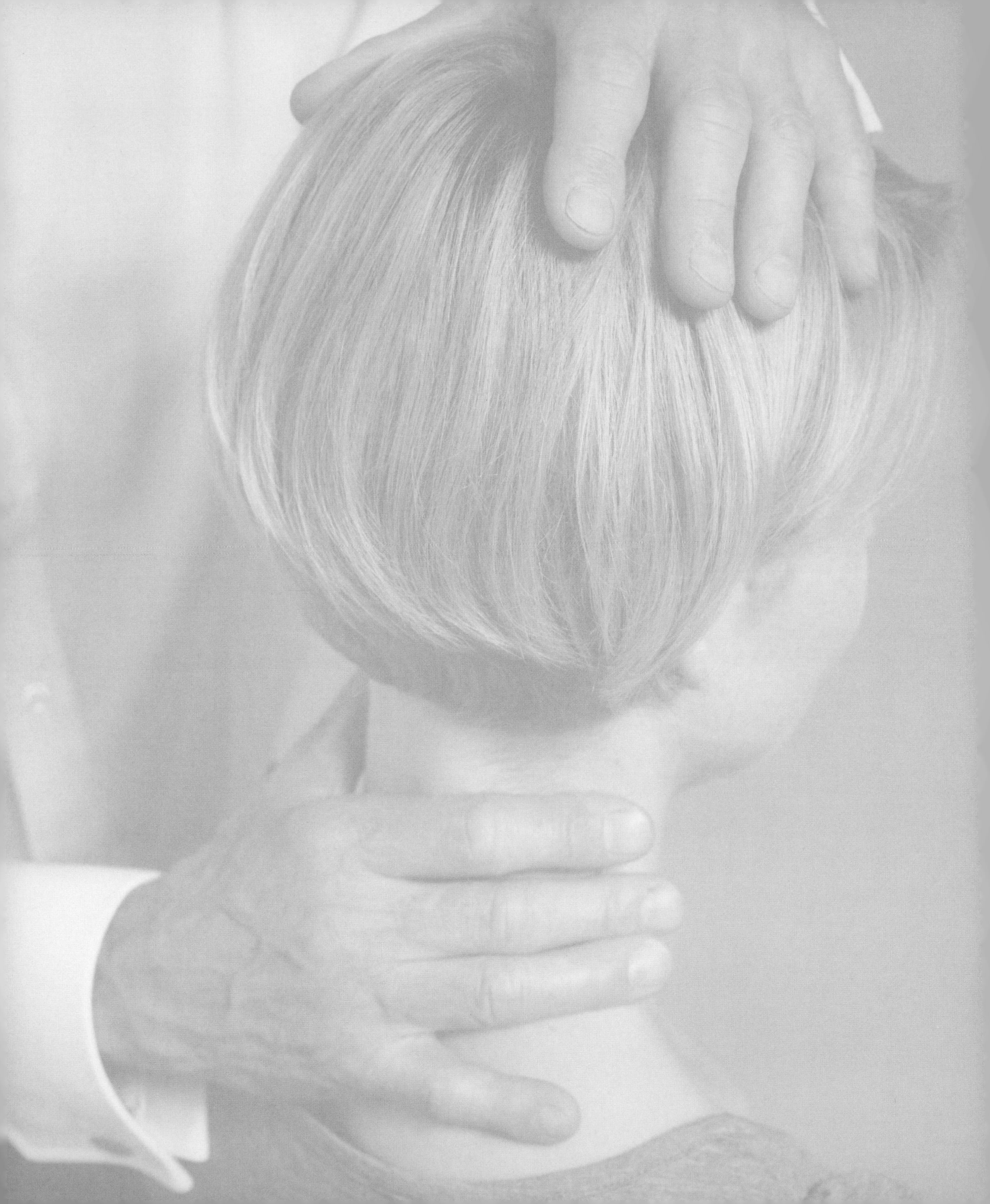

THE ALEXANDER TECHNIQUE

4

Psycho-physical unity

When it comes to ridding ourselves of back pain, it is a commonly held belief that there must be something wrong specifically with our back, so we seek treatment and do exercises to strengthen and increase mobility. However, it is unlikely that our back pain has anything more to do with our back than any other part of us; it's just that we feel the painful symptoms there. Any attempt to give treatment specifically to the painful area, or by strengthening the area, is unlikely to succeed if we do not take into consideration the manner in which we use our whole body during our daily life.

If we regularly hunch our shoulders or collapse into a slouch at our desk, there is so much of our body weight out of balance that it creates excessive strain throughout the body. Any treatment intended to cure back pain will barely tickle the surface of the problem.

Our body is not a collection of parts joined together but works as a whole; from the soles of our feet to the top of our head it works as one psycho-physical organism. This becomes more evident when we consider various activities of the body, such as the act of sitting. Is this an activity solely related to our back, or does it also involve our overall balance, the balance of our head, the support of our pelvis on the chair, muscle tone of our legs and whether our feet are on the floor? If we consider the process of digestion: is this solely a function of the digestive system, or does it also rely on the pumping of our heart to circulate adequate amounts of blood and the proper support of our torso to allow adequate space within our abdomen for the easy passage of food? Slouching can play havoc with our digestion and bowel movements.

Thinking is as much a physical function as it is a mental one as our brain relies on so much of our body to work efficiently. Where would our brain be without our heart to pump an oxygenated blood supply as well as a healthy body that digests food and is sufficiently mobile to carry our head around? If I send a text to a friend, is this purely a function of my hands, or does it also involve my arms and shoulders, my breathing, my back to support me and my digestion to nourish me as well as my mind? Our body would not function if it did not get the appropriate commands from our brain, consciously and subconsciously, through our various nervous systems. We can see that any activity we undertake involves our body and mind working together. Using the Alexander Technique involves our entire person, body and mind, and it brings about a more co-ordinated use of our whole.

The Alexander Technique is a form of psycho-physical re-education. It is the combined resource of body and mind, applying a 'means-whereby' approach, that re-educates our system.

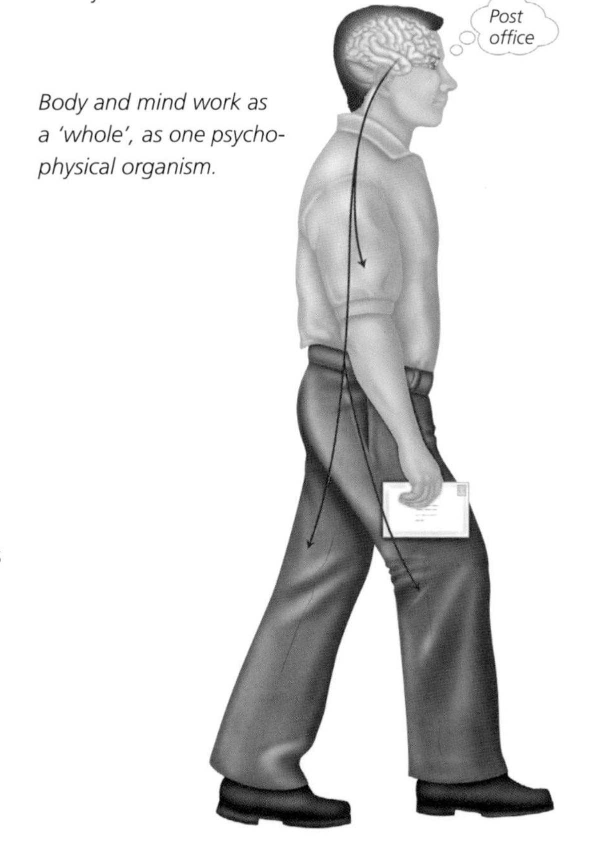

Body and mind work as a 'whole', as one psycho-physical organism.

Learning and using the Alexander Technique

Whether our reason for coming to the Alexander Technique is a painful back, stiff neck, stress, breathing problems or a wish for a better speaking voice and more confidence, the technique is applied in a very similar way. Although we may wish to rid ourselves of our painful symptoms, our approach needs to be an indirect one. Having eliminated other possible causes we now accept that back pain is due to poor posture, we will not work directly on the pain, but the overall cause of it.

Each and every one of us is unique with an infinitely varied range of tensions and postural habits that we have developed throughout our life. Having worked with thousands of people who have wanted to learn the Alexander Technique I have never met two the same, despite the fact that some may have complained of similar symptoms. The reason why the Alexander Technique will help each person in their own individual way is because the focus is to eliminate harmful habits. Regardless of why we may turn to the Alexander Technique, we need to bring our attention to the fundamental cause of our problems, which is our muscular co-ordination and balance. Whether it is a stiff neck, painful upper back, lower back, sciatic pain, or breathing problems, loss of voice or timidity and shyness, we need to address the inefficient co-ordination of our muscles that is causing poor functioning. If we attend to this, we will gain the improvements that we want, automatically and indirectly.

Those of us experienced in the Alexander Technique will seldom refer to posture, but rather to 'use'. The word posture implies positions that should be 'held', whereas in a healthy child they are free and constantly moving, using their physique in a well co-ordinated manner which is light, expansive and in balance. Postural habits tend to pull us off balance so we move with excessive tension and strain; we could then be described as having 'poor use'. How we 'use' ourselves governs how we function. If we bring our attention to 'how' we move and perform various activities, with a 'means-whereby' approach, we will bring about wonderfully free poise that encourages healthy working of the whole body. It is possible to develop 'good use' at any stage in our lives, if we bring our mind to it.

The Alexander Technique works because we are able to make choices about what we do and how we do it. Indeed we are the only species of vertebrate mammals able to make choices in this way. Alexander referred to our ability to move from subconscious to conscious guidance and control of ourselves, as 'man's supreme inheritance', the title of his first book.

The following pages outline how you can start thinking in order to inhibit harmful patterns and have more control over your 'use' so you make the most of yourself and eliminate back pain in the process!

Individual Alexander lessons

The Alexander Technique is normally learnt in the form of lessons from a qualified Alexander teacher who is likely to have completed a three-year full-time course involving over 1,600 hours of hands-on training. Their skill in observation and manual guidance will enable you to experience using your musculature in a different way. As F.M. Alexander discovered, we cannot sense accurately for ourselves what we are doing with our muscles and whether or not we are truly in balance. Our sensory perception is faulty due to the many years of habits affecting our co-ordination.

During the Alexander lesson you will perform various activities such as standing, sitting, walking and bending. The Alexander teacher will use their hands to gently guide you, so you get a new experience of being in better balance, freer in the joints and making less effort. You will also receive instruction on Inhibition and Direction so you become able to release unnecessary tensions while allowing yourself to come up to your full height and stature. You learn by experience and progress can be very quick, rewarding and enjoyable as the teacher can give accurate feedback throughout the lesson so you avoid possible problems. You learn how to think, to apply the principles of Inhibition and Direction for yourself, so you become self-sufficient.

A short initial course of 20–30 lessons is usually required, starting fairly intensively to help you to make the best possible progress. Further, less frequent, lessons may be desirable to help maintain your abilities and benefit you further.

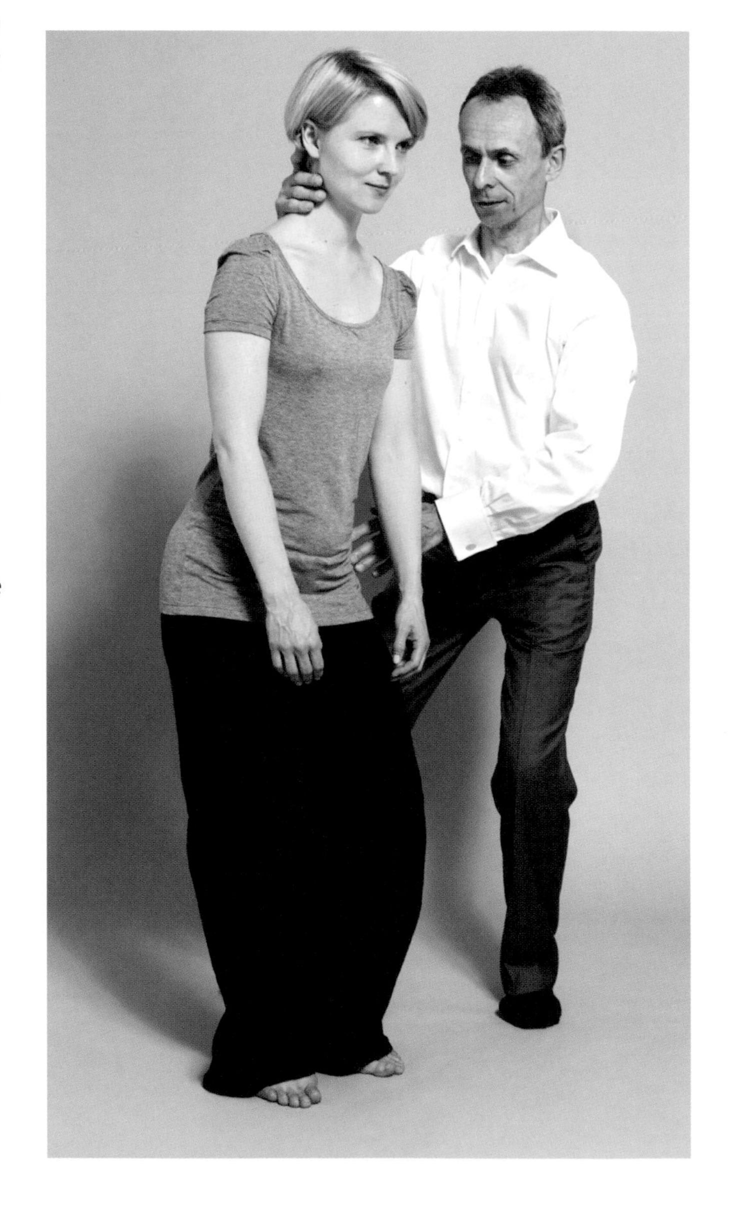

The teacher uses his hands very gently to help you release unnecessary tension and encourage a lengthening and widening of your stature. The new experience gradually becomes familiar.

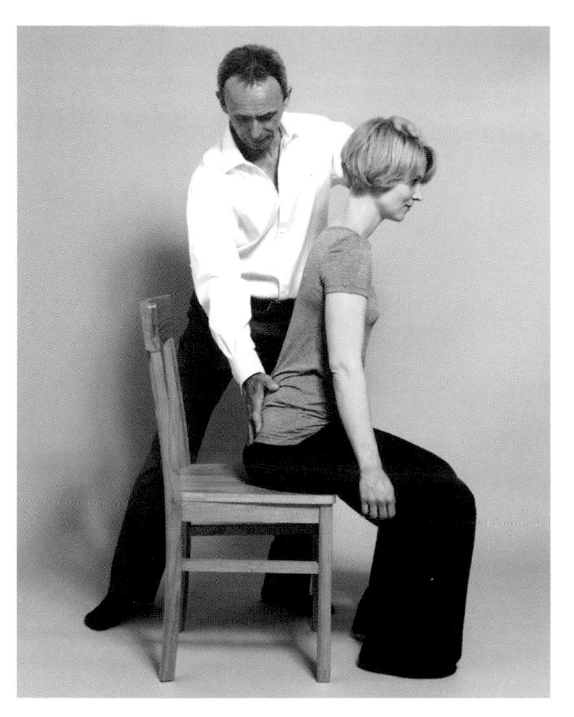

The hands-on guidance we receive during an Alexander lesson gives us a new sensory experience of making less effort and improved co-ordination.

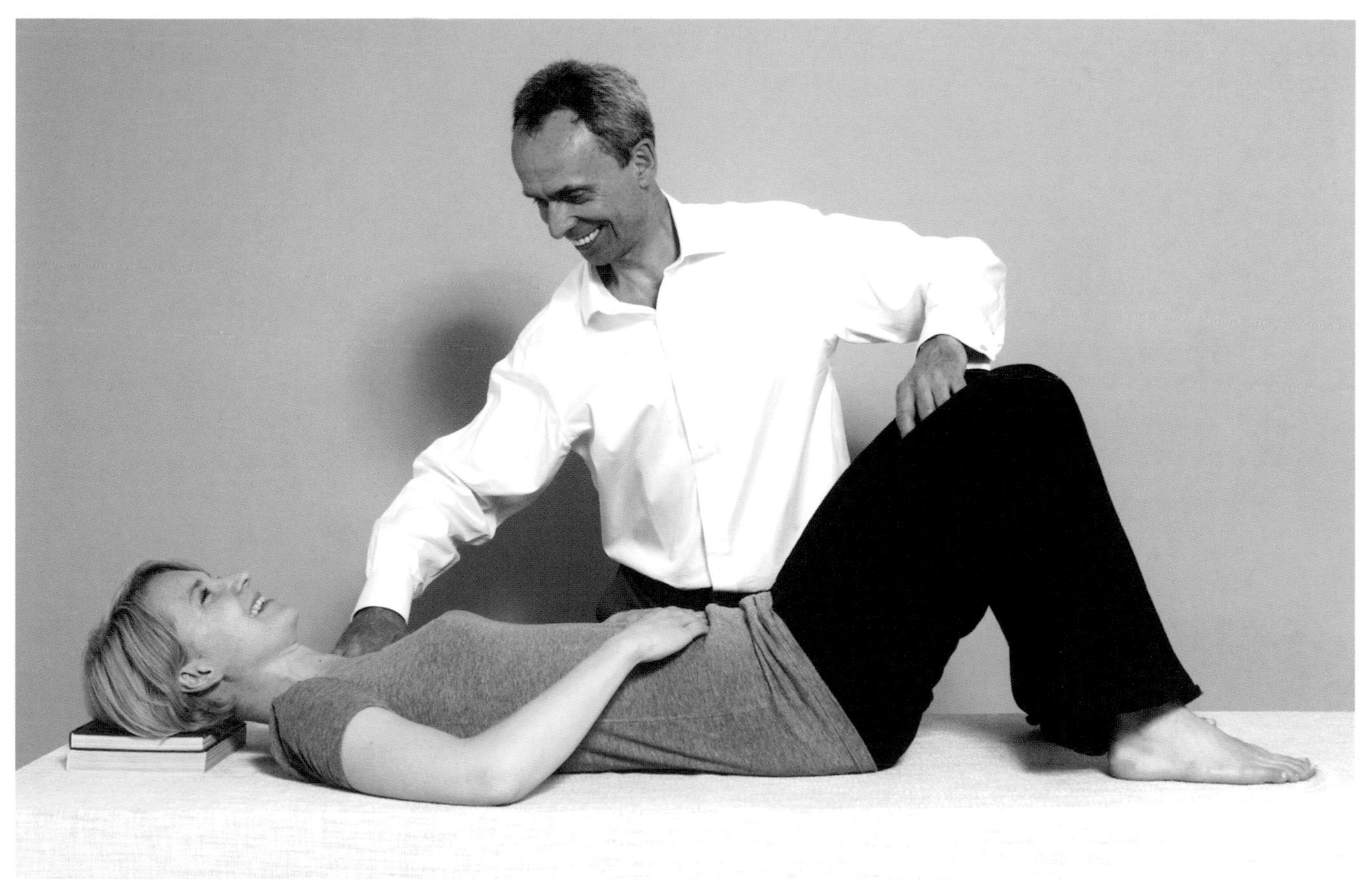

A thinking method

What a piece of work is a man! how noble in reason! how infinite in faculty! in form and moving how express and admirable! in action how like an angel! in apprehension how like a god! *Hamlet* by William Shakespeare

It is a commonly held belief that if we want to improve our poise and rid ourselves of back pain, we need to do something about it such as pull ourselves up straight. We may feel that we are not trying hard enough and some extra effort is required, but nothing could be further from the truth. Any effort to try and pull ourselves up tall, push our shoulders back or suck in our tummy will only cause extra tension and we will almost certainly use all the wrong muscles. This will create more discomfort and the development of further tensional habits that will further interfere with our poise. In other words, we will exchange one set of problems for another.

No matter what we may feel the problem is in relation to our poise, the actual cause is almost certainly muscular co-ordination and a misuse of our mechanisms. Our problems come about because we have some muscles making far too much effort, possibly continuously, and other muscles not doing enough. This is the cause of our bad back if all causes other than posture have been ruled out. It is our co-ordination that we need to change and this cannot be achieved by physically adjusting our position or making extra effort.

Healthy poise does not require any effort as our body 'knows' what to do. The cause of our problems is that we are now using our muscles differently from how we did when we enjoyed healthy poise as young children. We have all the muscles in the right place to do the job and we have an instinct for balance and poise inherited through the evolution of our species. The way to revive our natural poise is to get out of the way of ourselves and let it happen. We need to prevent old habits from kicking in and encourage better co-ordination. We need to allow our mechanisms to function as nature intended and this is achieved by our thinking and clear intention.

Does thinking work?

Thinking may be an activity of the brain, but from these thoughts, signals pass through the whole body. The brain is connected to the brainstem, the spinal cord and to every nerve ending in our body via the communication network of our nervous system. So for instance, if we think of food for a while, our mouth will begin to salivate and our tummy may rumble as digestive juices prepare to receive the food. The act of thinking constantly sends messages throughout the body causing different responses depending on the thoughts. The nerve pathways are always open. We do not need to worry about whether our thinking can have an effect, as it surely will. We use our 'thinking' with the Alexander Technique to release tension, lengthen and widen, and although results may not be instant, we must inhibit trying to force any change; the messages will get through.

As an individual you have potentially far more control and influence over your body and health than anyone else. Using your thinking to change your health and well-being may seem strange at first, but you soon get used to it and are likely to benefit in ways beyond your imagination.

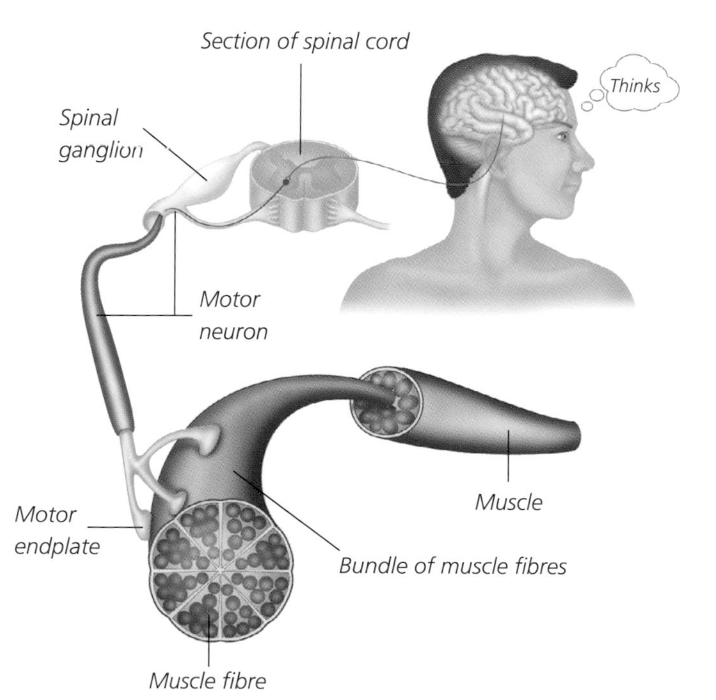

It involves no effort

The Alexander Technique is a thinking technique that requires no physical effort. Of course muscles will be working otherwise we'd end up in a heap on the floor, but there will be no sense of effort if they are working in a well co-ordinated manner.

We make changes to our co-ordination by thinking. It involves thinking certain thoughts which combine to overcome poor habits and bring about an improved manner of use. With so many hundreds of muscles in our body, they all need to work together in a well-synchronised fashion, much as they did when we were habit-free toddlers. Now as adults we have some muscles working too hard, causing tension, shortening and compression of our body, while other muscles are not doing enough and remaining flaccid. We need all of our muscles to work together, each doing their fair share of the work – not too much and not too little – so that the appropriate amount of effort is used throughout our whole body for any particular activity.

The quality that we require is expansive in stature so we sit and stand at our full height and width; we want to be in continuous good balance so we are free in all of our joints and expending the minimum of effort. This is the quality we require to avoid strain and help ourselves function healthily. The first consideration is to inhibit the harmful tensions that interfere with our natural upright poise.

Our brain is in constant communication with our muscles via the nervous system.

Unreliable sensory appreciation

In the last chapter we experimented with changing the way in which we stood or sat and how wrong it felt to stand differently. We have been engaging in these habits for so long that they feel right; like a worn-out pair of shoes that needs replacing, they feel comfortable even if they are causing harm. This shows how our habits have affected the accuracy of our sensory appreciation (kinaesthetic sense). But there is no possibility that we can know what is right if we go by our feelings that are so clearly wrong. Any change we may make to the way we sit, stand or move is therefore likely to feel wrong because it does not fit with our faulty sensory appreciation.

It was while endeavouring to overcome his own vocal and postural problems by using mirrors for feedback about his poise that F.M. Alexander discovered his own faulty sensory appreciation. He realised that habits affect our sensory appreciation to the degree that our awareness provides less than reliable feedback about our condition and poise.

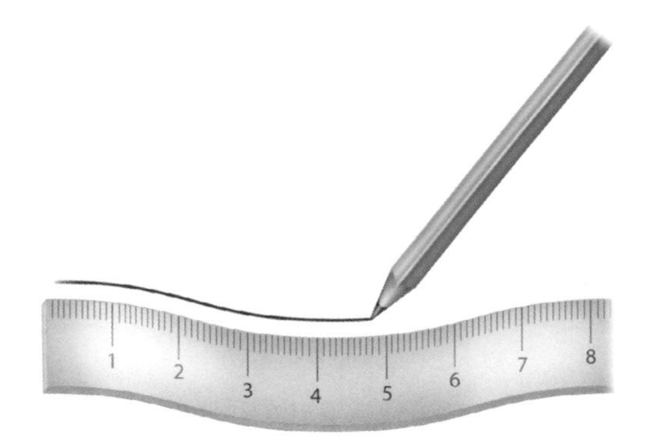

You can't know a thing by an instrument that is wrong.

F. M. Alexander

He concluded that since he could not rely on his feelings to guide him, he must rely on observation and the mirror reflection to tell him what he was doing. He realised that his faulty sensory perception would not guide him to know if he was right or wrong, and he eventually learnt to rely on his technique of 'inhibition' and 'direction' to bring about the correct working of his mechanisms, even if the sensation felt wrong. Through his experimentation over a period of time he changed his whole manner of use and his sensory awareness also improved. Today we have Alexander teachers who provide accurate feedback about our poise during lessons. Sensory Motor Learning re-trains our overall co-ordination so our kinaesthetic sense improves.

End-gaining

In today's hurly-burly lifestyle we are so focused on achieving results, matching up to expectations, delivering on schedule, passing exams and getting the job done that we rarely give any attention to *how* we are achieving them. F.M. Alexander referred to the tendency of only having the end result in sight as 'end-gaining'. When we are in this mode, the manner in which we perform the task does not even enter our consciousness, so we suffer the consequences of our habits.

To do list ...

Walk dog

Shopping

Pick up dry cleaning

An aching back is often painful proof and evidence of the postural habits we have adopted during our lives. Accepting that our muscular co-ordination is not as finely tuned as we might like, that we are probably not in good balance most of the time and that we also create more or less exertion than required for any given task means it is likely that we will display all these undesirable qualities in everything we do. Our actions are characterised by our habits, unless we inhibit them. With each and every repetition of our habits, they become more ingrained and more pronounced, becoming more evident as we get older.

Applying a 'means-whereby' approach, or non-end-gaining, means giving attention to how we perform activities. We will still achieve our objectives but do so with far less strain and wear and tear on the body as well as conserving more energy.

Non-end-gaining is an indirect approach to doing activities while looking after ourselves in the process. For example, if

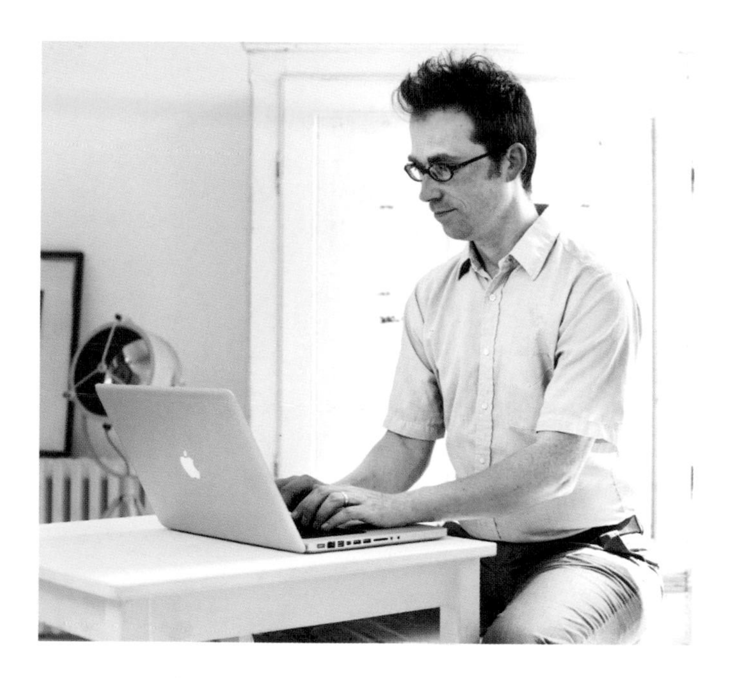

we are aware of how we are typing, we would gently tap the keyboard of our computer rather than hammering it in such a way that we are sure to end up with Repetitive Strain Injury.

By inhibiting our instinctive reaction to rush ahead we give ourselves time to work on the 'means-whereby' rather than the end result. We can do our task while avoiding the pitfalls of our habits and stop the interference that gets in the way of healthy poise. Remember, the right thing will do itself if we let it. When learning a new skill such as playing the piano, guitar or golf, we learn to consciously control *how* we are functioning so we can bring the best from ourselves. We should apply a 'means-whereby' approach to all our activities and let the result take care of itself.

Inhibition

The word inhibition in the Alexander Technique sense has very positive connotations and no connection to Freud's theory of repression. Inhibition helps us bring about change to virtually every aspect of our being. Far from being restrictive, it helps us avoid reacting to stimuli in a stereotyped manner characterised by a lifetime's habits and can actually allow our natural spontaneity to emerge. Fundamentally, inhibiting allows us to employ a 'means-whereby' approach to our activities so we can choose *how* we do them. We often use the word inhibition in subtly different ways:

1. To inhibit our response to stimuli.
2. To inhibit 'doing' – allow time to stop.
3. To inhibit postural habits.
4. To inhibit reacting to the desire to change your posture by using force or effort (end-gaining).

To inhibit our response to stimuli

There are so many demands being made on our time and constant stimuli inundating our senses that we become extremely reactive. Most of us react to ideas and external stimuli without stopping to think about our poise or how to avoid the effect of our harmful postural habits. For example, when the phone rings we instantly pick it up; if we want to get a bag from another room we instantly rise from the chair, go into the room and when we pick up our bag, we do so without a second thought about how we are likely stiffening harmfully and collapsing our back. We are 'end-gaining'. Most of the things we do during the day are conducted by instant reactions to a signal, command or thought, but seldom do we consider how we are performing the movement. For example, in what manner we are bending down or picking up the phone. If we stop for a moment before reacting, we may even decide not to act at all. Stopping gives us time to make a choice about what we do and how we do it.

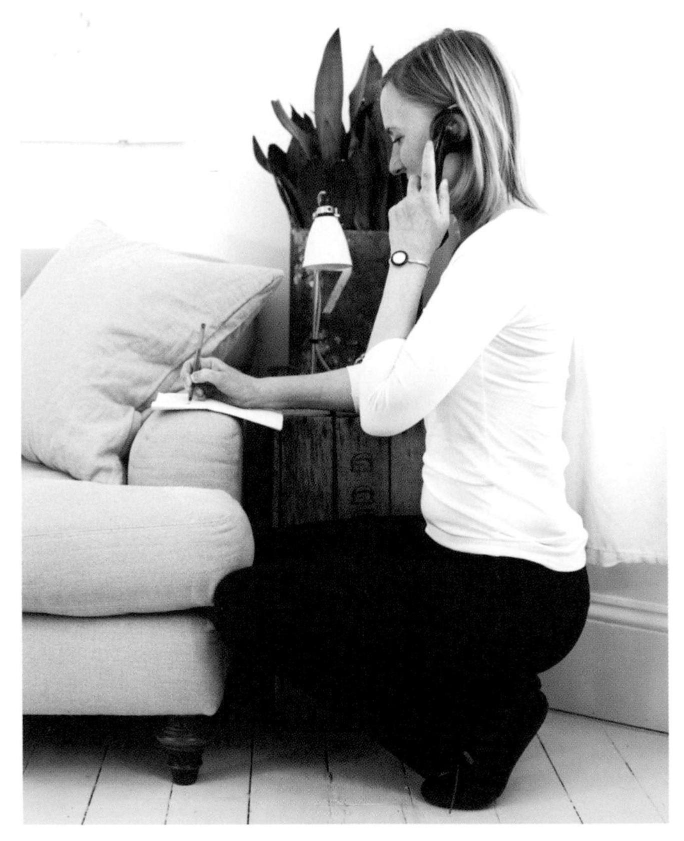

Taking time gives you a chance to choose how you move.

If we are going to avoid habitual tensions from occurring and avoid pain as we bend or reach for something, or indeed change how we use ourselves during any activity, we need

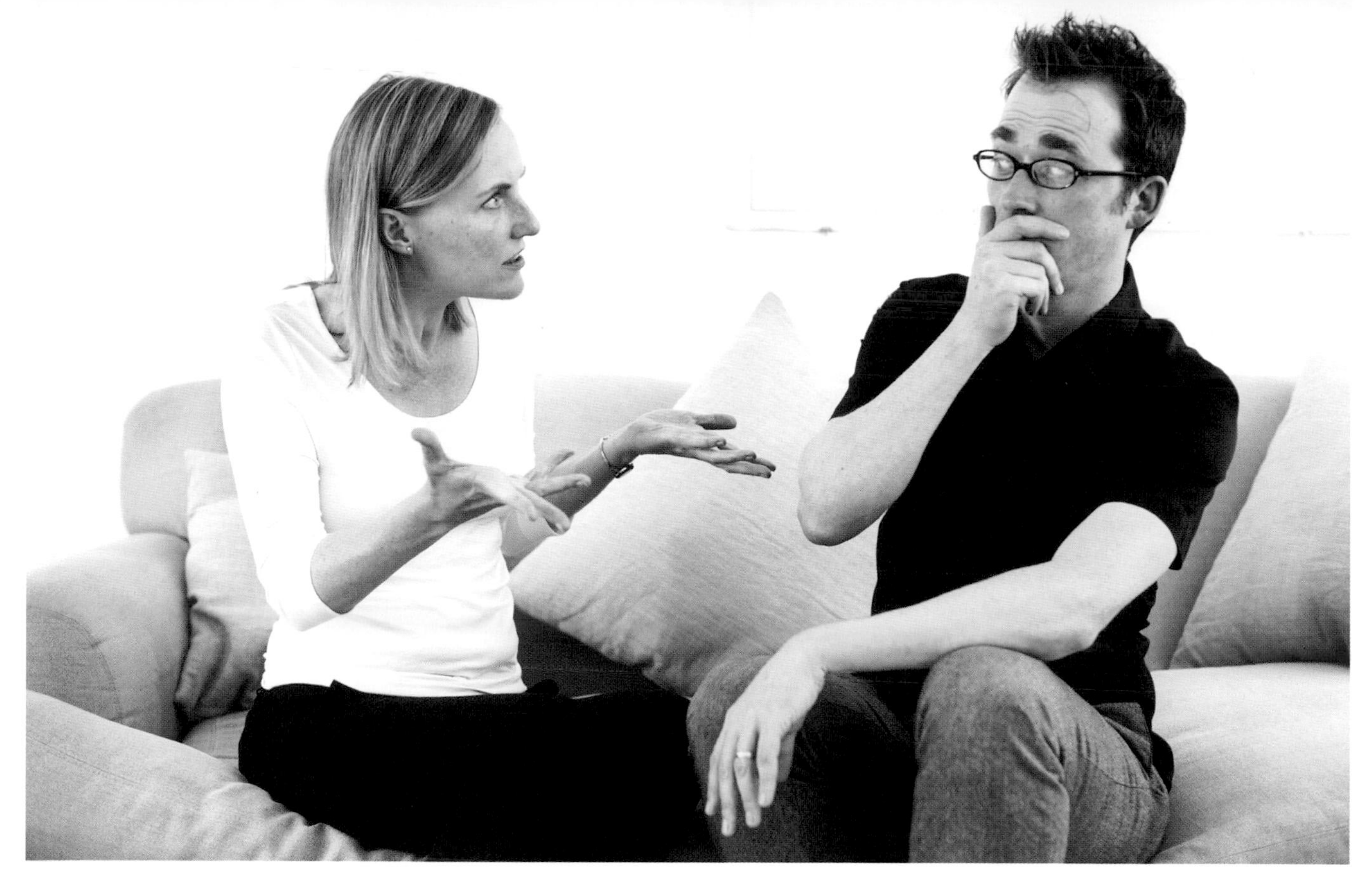

"I wish I hadn't said that!" – Inhibiting first lets you choose the best way of saying something or performing a task.

to give ourselves time to think; we need to 'inhibit', to stop and give ourselves just a moment. If we instantly react to a stimulus, we do not allow ourselves that opportunity and consequently our habits become ingrained. By stopping to think before we reach for the phone, for instance, we give ourselves the chance to release tension in our neck and to reach out with the minimum of effort, causing the least strain to our back while expending the least amount of effort possible. By inhibiting we give ourselves the chance of using a 'means-whereby' approach which allows us to react with greater consciousness about how and what we do.

Inhibition can also play a positive role socially; instead of reacting emotionally in stressful situations we can pause for a second or two before responding in a calmer and more considered way.

The process of giving ourselves time should not be a luxury afforded to rare occasions but needs to become a way of life. We will get just as much done in the day if not more.

By giving ourselves just a second or two to think, we can allow ourselves the chance to behave and move as we would wish. How many times have you said to yourself, 'I wish I'd thought more about that before I did it!'?

Pausing to think before reacting ('non-end-gaining') is helpful in so many ways: we become more considered in our actions and words and less reactive, we create less adrenalin and become less stressed, our breathing may become slower and more regular, we make fewer mistakes by not rushing and we prevent unnecessary tensions from interfering with the fluidity and ease of our movement.

Inhibiting gives us time to apply the Alexander Technique directions, as explained in the next section. Inhibition means stop. By stopping or pausing first to think before reacting, we give ourselves the chance to consider how we move. It may take only a second, but by this means we begin to change our lives. This is fundamental to the Alexander Technique and without it no progress will be made.

To inhibit 'doing' – allow time to stop

Most of us experience life as being fairly busy and for many, it's totally hectic. We rush from one activity to another, thinking of two things at once as our mind works overtime. This manner of conducting ourselves can be very stressful and quite damaging. If every day is similar and we are constantly on the go, it is likely that when we sit down in the evening, we just collapse in front of the TV. But this 'busy-ness' can also become an internal condition. Our psycho-physical mechanism can become very 'busy' even when doing nothing. So if we ever sit down, possibly in a train, taxi, bus or café, we may still be very 'active' inside; our brain may be working on a myriad of things and the musculature of our neck, shoulders, arms and legs can all be tensing in a form of constant agitation. This condition of internal restlessness, fidgeting, twitching and generally over revving of ourselves as though we are stuck in the equivalent of third gear, is not a good condition to be in, and can lead to high blood pressure, heart disease and other internal disorders. We need to slow down inside.

Whenever we can, we should stop 'doing' and stop 'thinking' for a while to give ourselves time to unwind. We can bring our conscious mind to our situation, sitting or standing somewhere, empty our mind of all the urgent things and allow an air of stillness to pervade us. We can become more aware of our breathing, allowing it to slow and deepen. We can relax our neck, hands and arms, and stop fidgeting with our legs and feet by letting them rest on the floor. Release unnecessary tensions; calm and quieten our body and mind.

And we must ensure that when we begin to give Alexander Technique 'directions', we are not trying to overlay or superimpose these on top of our internal restlessness. By seeking greater calmness and stillness of body and mind, we are putting ourselves more into a condition of neutrality, which is a most helpful basis on which to build our abilities with the technique.

However it should be noted before we begin learning the Alexander Technique that it is not always possible for us to achieve as much 'stillness' within us as we might like. So I would like to reassure you that by learning and beginning to apply the technique, you are likely to discover that you become quieter inside anyway. You will find that the technique promotes greater calmness and stillness. This becomes self-fulfilling if we allow it, as the internal quietness that we experience with the Alexander Technique will enable us to stop more easily to find greater quietness and calmness.

To inhibit postural habits

As our body works as a whole, it is not possible to eliminate back pain caused by the loss of natural poise without addressing balance and co-ordination.

Postural habits become ingrained over many years of practice and consequently we are unaware of them. But if we stop to pay attention to ourselves we may discover that we are tightening our shoulders or pulling back our head by stiffening our neck. Such tensional habits are unnecessary and unwanted. We need to inhibit them to prevent them from affecting our poise and movement.

Try to notice any little tensions that exist that may be unnecessary. Are your ankles wrapped around the chair as you sit? Inhibit this tendency and put your feet flat on the floor. Are you holding your head on one side continuously? Inhibit the muscle tension in one side of your neck and allow

> Everyone is always teaching one what to do, leaving us still doing things we shouldn't do. F. M. Alexander

your head to balance centrally. (We will discuss this in greater detail further on in this chapter.) Are you holding your breath? Inhibit this and allow your breathing to recommence freely and easily; inhibit blowing or sucking... just let it happen. Are you holding one shoulder higher than the other? Inhibit this and allow it to drop downward; inhibit pulling it downward. See if you can just let it release.

Tension can exist whether we are simply sitting or standing still and this unnecessary muscle activity burns energy and causes deterioration and stress. If we liken our situation to driving a car, it would be as though we were sitting stationary at traffic lights with the clutch depressed while revving the engine at 4,000rpm. It serves no purpose, wastes fuel and causes wear and tear on the moving parts. Whenever possible we should put ourselves into a condition of 'neutral' and not 'rev' ourselves all the time, emotionally or physically.

To inhibit reacting to the desire to change your posture by using force or effort

When we wish to make changes to our posture, the desire to see results of our endeavours can be so great that we may instinctively try too hard. Giving a 'helping hand' by making a little effort forms a significant part of what Alexander referred to as 'end-gaining' (see page 63). Don't. Just because you cannot feel anything happening when you are thinking of releasing or directing, doesn't mean nothing is happening; subtle changes may be taking place as a result of your thinking of which you are as yet unaware. Inhibit your tendency to make an effort as no effort is required or wanted. This is the way it works. It is very much about doing nothing and all about thinking.

You will only discover if it works by following these guidelines and giving it time; your teacher will be able to guide you in your thinking. If you are reading this book and applying the principles for the first time, it's important to adhere to the guidelines. The next section will show you how to think, so you can revive the quality of freedom and expansiveness in your poise.

Inhibition is the cornerstone of the Alexander Technique. It is only by inhibiting our responses to stimuli, inhibiting our tensional habits and inhibiting our tendency to try too hard that we can we make changes to our co-ordination. Remember it is our co-ordination that needs to change first and changes in our posture will follow automatically. We can only do this by thinking.

> He gets what he feels is the right position, but when he has an imperfect co-ordination he is only getting in a position which fits with his defective co-ordination. F. M. Alexander

Muscle memory

Muscle memory plays a major part in everything we do. If it wasn't for muscle memory, we would never get past the beginning stages of learning a new skill. It's muscle memory that we rely on when we write, so we do not need to think about the dexterity required to hold a pen, touch-type the keys on a Qwerty keyboard, play the piano, tie our shoe laces or knot our tie. By repetition of an action the muscles involved record patterns of tension in relation to one another – i.e. the co-ordination of muscles required to do the job – so after a few practices we can achieve the movements without thinking. Muscle memory is most helpful in virtually everything we do, however it does not discriminate between accurate and good muscle use and badly co-ordinated poor muscle use: it picks it all up in equal measure. It's a double-edged sword – we can develop bad postural habits just as quickly as we can develop good ones.

By acting instinctively and 'end-gaining' in all that we do, we ingrain our habits; we practise and reinforce our mistakes as well as our successes! When learning any new skill, we should first choose a good example to copy, for example Yehudi Menuhin playing the violin, Tiger Woods swinging a golf club, Venus Williams playing tennis, Arthur Rubinstein poised at the piano and anyone else you consider to display ultimate perfection in the act of performing. To learn how to bend without straining your back, watch a two-year-old child! When learning a new skill, look closely at how your mentor uses himself or herself and set up good habits from the outset by copying their use. This may involve slowing your movements right down or even breaking the movements into smaller sections that you can practise slowly and carefully so the positive experience is stored in your muscle memory. Eventually you can speed up and join the various parts of a movement together so you instil good co-ordination free of poor habits.

With the Alexander Technique we learn to think as we move. We learn to inhibit harmful tensions and ensure healthy free and fluid movements, all the while maintaining good balance. Each and every time we repeat a good experience such as sitting well with a free, lengthening and widening back in good balance, it's reinforced in our subconscious and we develop good and healthy manner of use.

By using the Alexander Technique we give maximum attention to the manner in which we perform movements, how we sit, stand, walk and bend to ensure we minimise poor habits and weaken the muscle memory of unhelpful habits while instilling muscle memory of good 'use' and improved co-ordination.

Arthur Rubinstein displayed wonderful natural poise, on and off the concert stage. Good poise needs to be a part of us generally for it to be available when peak performance is required.

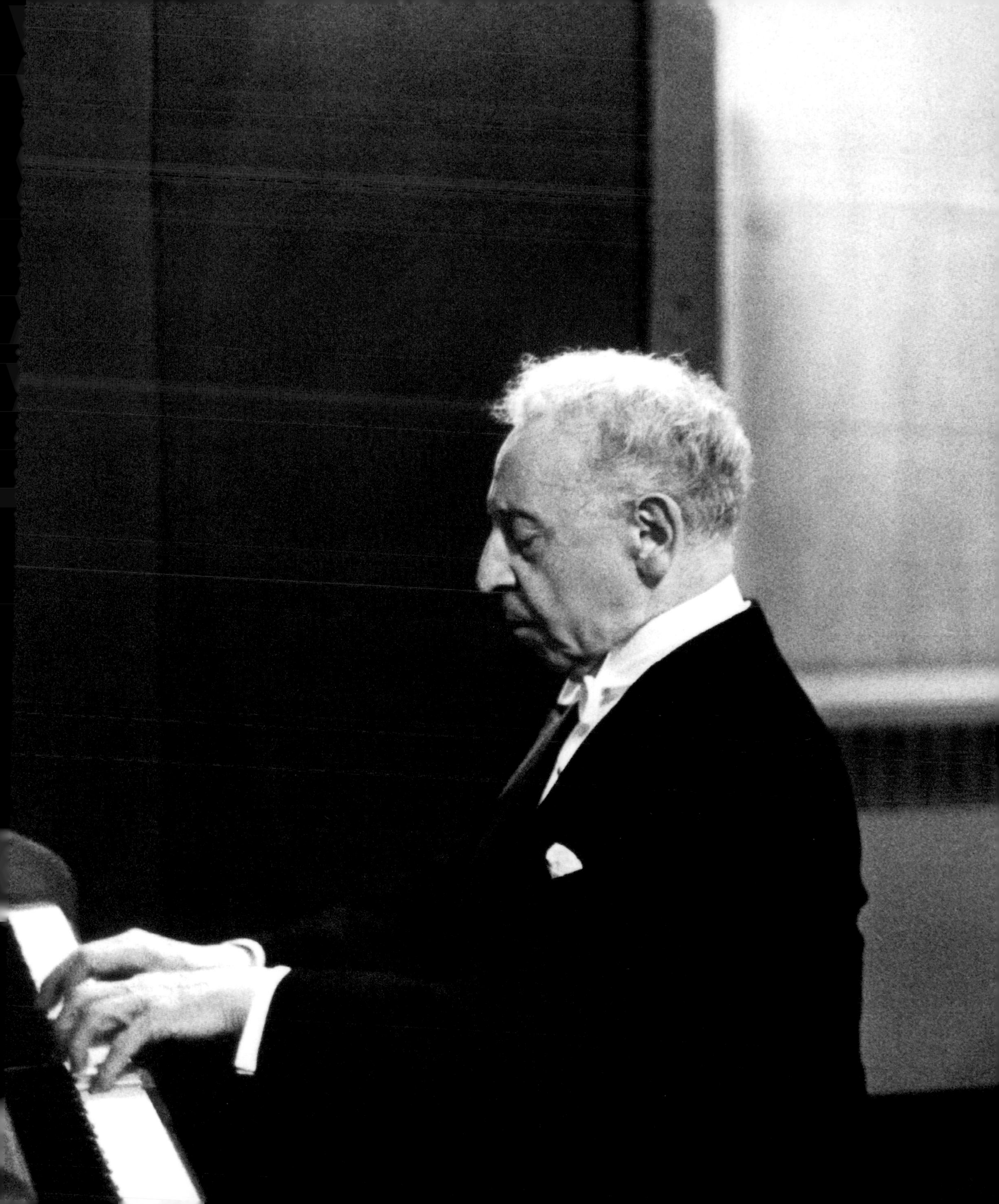

How to think to release unnecessary tension

Postural habits tend to involve an excess of muscular tension. At any given time there will also be other muscles which are underactive and we will discuss how we can activate them in a well co-ordinated manner when we look at Direction in the next section.

If we've been working out and playing a great deal of sport, certain muscle groups may become over-contracted as a consequence of the unfamiliar level of use and activity. Doing warm-up and cool-down stretches will help avoid injury and prevent muscles from becoming locked up. Consult your physical trainer for expert guidance in this matter.

With the Alexander Technique we learn how to release unnecessary habitual tension by thought. To release unwanted tension, we can think of the area involved as softening, melting and releasing. These words mean much the same thing and really it's whatever works for you that matters. *Allow* your muscles to release. By thinking of melting or letting go, we encourage the muscles within a given area to release their unwanted contractions. We may not feel the release in a specific area immediately as it can take a few moments. Deeper release of tension may come later if we continue asking for the release in our mind. It is worthwhile sticking with the thought of 'letting go' for several moments and even minutes. If you think you've achieved it, then ask for it again.

Muscles will tend to return to habitual patterns even though they may have released. When this happens it's best not to have an 'end-gaining' attitude, 'ticking the box' when we've released and getting on with something else. Consider releasing as an on-going activity. It is the search for the release that is important, not the finding it. If you think you've found the freedom you were looking for, throw it away and look for it again. An ongoing attitude to release gradually retrains the muscles.

The experience you want is in the process of getting it. If you have something, give it up. Getting it, not having it, is what you want. F.M. Alexander

An inquisitive and explorative approach to allowing the release of tension is a better frame of mind to encourage deeper changes rather than simply superficial ones. Enquire within given areas for different ways of letting go. Stick with it for minutes if you can. Even when we are relaxed, repeating the instruction helps prevent habits creeping in.

Lying in Semi-supine Position (described on page 98) is an excellent way of helping to release unnecessary tensions, revive tired muscles and restore free and upright poise. It's wonderful for helping to relieve an aching back.

Releasing tension in our neck is such an important aspect of poise we shall be looking at this in considerable detail. Directing ourselves to 'lengthen' and 'widen' helps release unnecessary muscle tension too and we will be considering this in the next section.

Exercise – Releasing 1

›› We can all make a fist briefly so that we tighten those muscles and then let them relax. But you are now going to experiment with asking for more release of tension than is your normal state.

›› Place your hand on a table, or your knee if you are sitting, with your palm facing upward. Allow it to soften, let your fingers go limp and free, allow the palm of your hand to open and spread. You are now releasing unnecessary tension. Do this for 30 seconds or so. Sense your hand releasing and opening out. If you feel that it did let go, well done. But don't stop there, think of releasing more; give it more time. Ask your hand to lengthen and widen. Give it a couple of minutes. Now you're searching beyond the superficial. Work on the process of letting go and forget the end result (see page 94).

Exercise – Releasing 2

›› Sit at a table and put your hand out so that it lies palm flat on the table. Notice if your elbow is sticking out to the side. If so, can you allow your elbow to drop, by means of its own weight and gravity? Is your shoulder raised too? Can you let it drop? Think of it softening.

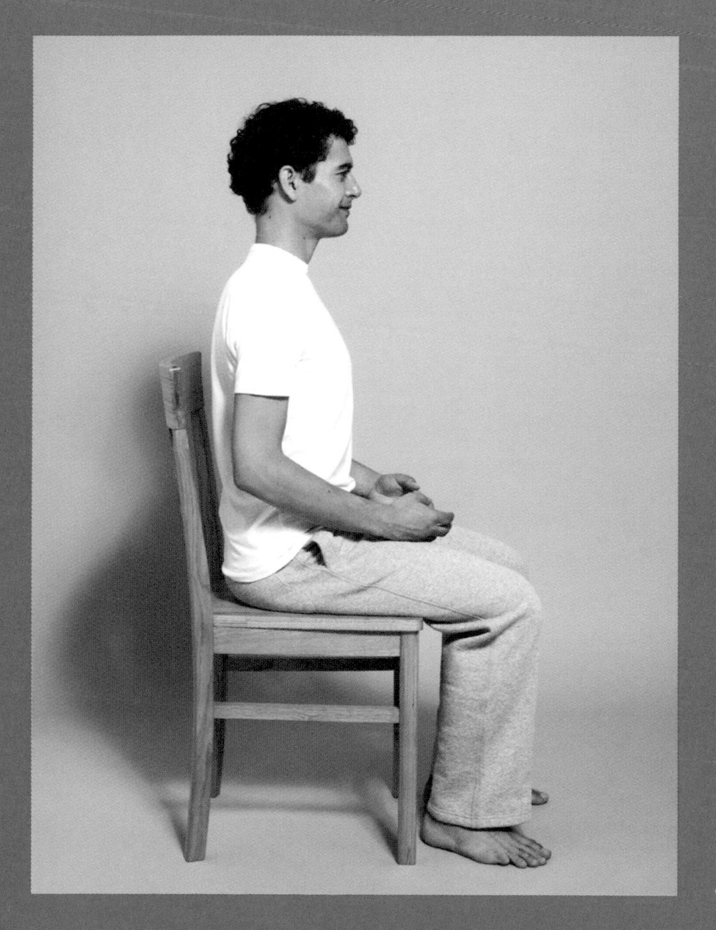

Exercise – Releasing 3

›› While sitting, place your feet flat on the floor in front of you. Notice, are your feet absolutely flat on the floor or are your heels held upward? If they are not flat, think of your hips releasing, your upper leg softening and going downward and allow your heel to drop onto the floor. Do not push it, just allow it to release.

When sitting, allow your weight to go through your sitting bones and allow your legs and arms to release.

Directions

The Alexander Technique is often mistakenly considered a relaxation technique, but if all we did was relax and release tension we would soon fall to the floor in a heap. To help our body to function well and enjoy healthy poise, we need our muscles to work, and to do so in a well co-ordinated manner.

If 'inhibition' is a way of giving ourselves time to think and prevent tension habits from affecting our poise, the giving of directions is how we further release unnecessary tension as well as energise our muscles and bring about a healthy co-ordination in our back and throughout the whole body. No matter what reason we have for learning the Alexander Technique, be it back pain, breathing or voice problems, it is the co-ordinated use of ourselves that determines how we function. It is no use just pulling ourselves up 'straight' or pulling our shoulders back as this only creates further tension that will cause other problems; by so doing we're only pulling ourselves around and meddling with an extremely complex mechanism. We can enhance our co-ordination by using a combination of Inhibition and Direction. They work together. We 'inhibit' to give ourselves time to think, we 'inhibit' our harmful habits and we 'direct' to release tensions and improve our co-ordination. Moment by moment we 'inhibit' and 'direct'; they go hand in hand.

Giving directions is the thought process of sending commands, or 'Orders', from our brain to our body's mechanisms. They do not involve any effort, but rely purely on a mental command that is rather in the form of a wish, desire or clear intention. However the thought is not a daydream; we must intend it to happen. It does not require severe concentration, which might furrow our brow, just the clear wish – and this will bring about the correct working of our mechanisms.

We give ourselves directions to release unnecessary contractions and lengthen and widen in stature. The cumulative effect is to improve the working of our back so that it functions expansively, supporting us as we move around with suppleness and flexibility. The quality that we will bring about is exactly what happens in nature, not only in our children but also in other vertebrate mammals such as cats, lions, dogs, horses and cheetahs. Bearing in mind that we all have an instinct for healthy poise and functioning, we must not 'try' to do it, our body knows what to do, we just need to give it the instructions and allow it to respond.

When an investigation comes to be made, it will be found that every single thing we are doing in the work is exactly what is being done in Nature where the conditions are right, the difference being that we are learning to do it consciously. F. M. Alexander

The directions we give with the Alexander Technique do not isolate any particular muscle or muscle group but co-ordinate many muscles to work collectively in a well-synchronised manner. It is a condition that will bring about the best 'use' of ourselves and prevent back pain.

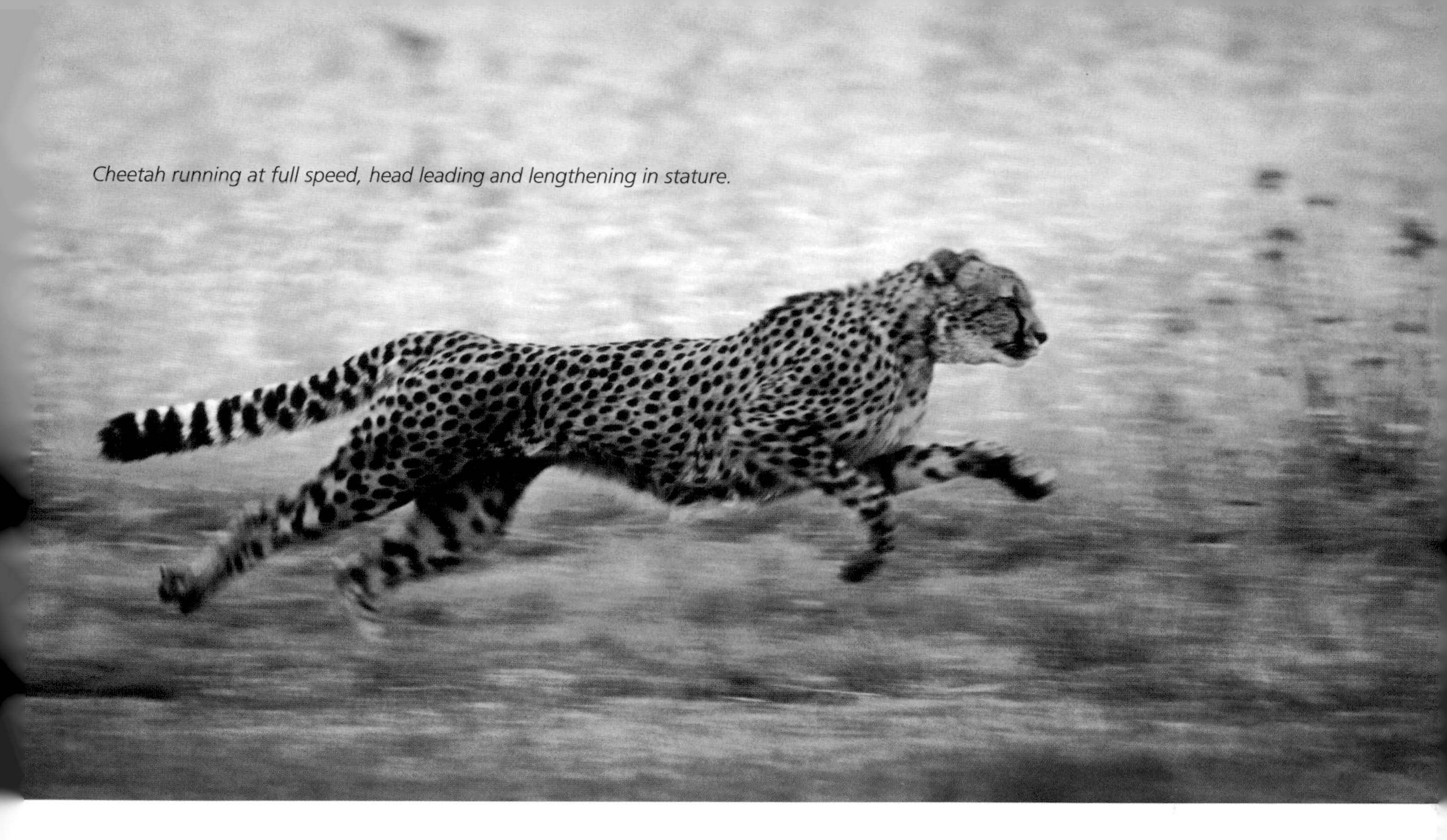

Cheetah running at full speed, head leading and lengthening in stature.

The quality we want is one of being very free in all our joints and expansive, just as we were as children. The directions we give tap into our instinct and revive this quality.

Being free and expansive in stature is a very large concept and beyond our ability to bring about in one fell swoop. So Alexander evolved a series of principle Directions that cumulate to bring about this quality and we do so by attending to one step at a time. We will apply these directions as a 'means-whereby' we can change our poise. It is a step-by-step process. They apply whether we are standing, sitting or lying down in 'Semi-supine'. Each direction is thought in turn, but we keep each one going as we add the next, one after the other and progressively all together.

The Primary Directions are:

1. **Neck to be free**
2. **Head to go forward and up**
3. **Back to lengthen**
4. **Back to widen**
5. **Knees to go forward and away**

(Note: It is crucially important to remember that these directions are thoughts and require no effort. If we simply attempt to pull ourselves up straight or push our head forward and upward we would tighten muscles which would be counter-productive. We must remember that our first consideration is not to try and change our posture or get rid of back pain, although those ideas may be in the back of our mind. By using the Alexander Technique, we rely on the 'means-whereby' approach of thinking in order to change the co-ordination of our muscles. This needs to be our only consideration and wish, and we do it by thinking. If you believe otherwise, you must change your thinking so that this becomes your priority, otherwise it won't work. The Alexander Technique is a thinking method to change our muscle co-ordination; if we improve our co-ordination we bring about the correct working of our body and our posture will change accordingly.)

1. Neck to be free

Allowing the neck to be free plays a crucial role in co-ordinating the whole body, so we enjoy better poise and help avoid back pain.

There are seven cervical vertebrae and a great many muscles in the neck, all involved in supporting and moving our head. The co-ordination of these muscles is very important, not only for the neck, but also for the healthy working of the whole body. However, in terms of improving our poise, we are particularly interested in helping our head to balance freely on the top-most vertebra of the spine called the Atlas.

Most of us have enormous strength in our neck as a consequence of a lifetime of tensing the muscles; indeed it is far stronger than it need be for normal living. If we look at young children around 2–3 years old, they have very large heads for the relative size of their body and very slim necks and their heads balance very freely on top of their spine. At that age they do not have the strength to stiffen their muscles, so their head 'teeters' and balances very freely. Indeed if a 14-month-old toddler who is just learning to stand lets their head go backward off balance, they will fall over onto their bottom. As adults we develop such strength in our neck that we can hold our head in an off-balance position all day. But this has a significant effect on our overall balance and can contribute to such problems as headaches, stiff necks, aching back, poor breathing and other internal dysfunction and stress. Good head balance and a free neck are crucial for healthy poise and good co-ordination.

When we stiffen our neck, we are mostly tightening the muscles around the back of the head. This is linked to the 'startle pattern' or 'flight or fight' reflex (see page 22). Constantly holding on to stress eventually leads to degenerative disorders such as arthritis as well as poor breathing, general stiffness, neck and back pain. By using the Alexander Technique we address the situation and break the cycle so we lose our 'startle pattern' posture and become more upright and calm.

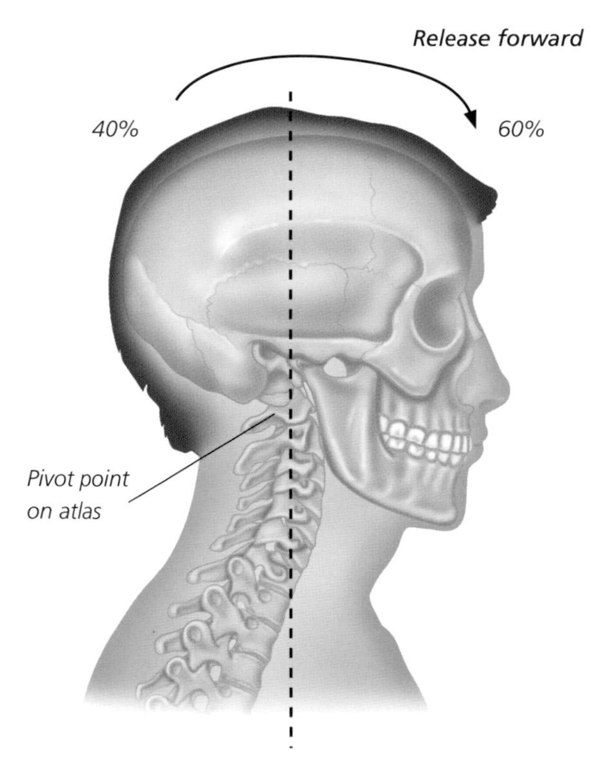

Head weight is greater in front of the Atlas.

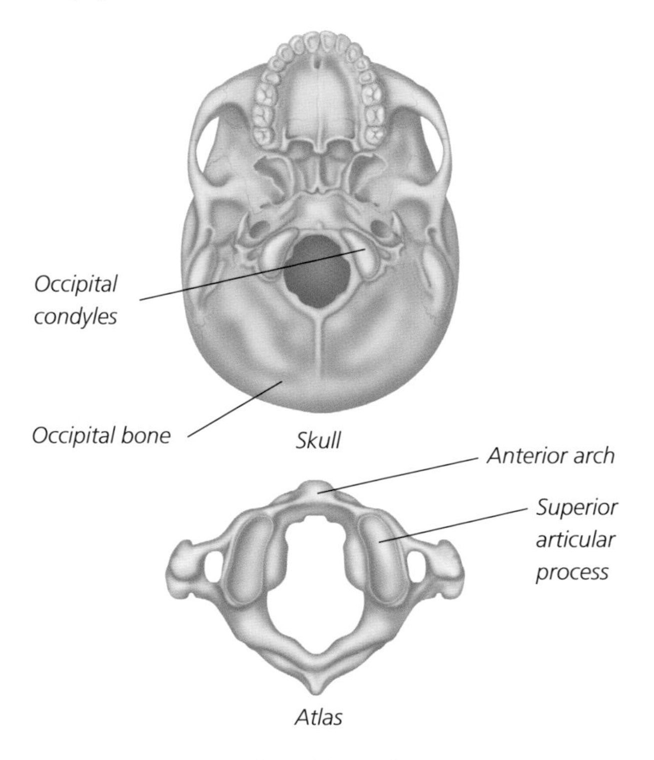

The occipital condyles under the skull sit into the processes of the Altlas.

HEAD BALANCE

The skull balances on the top vertebra of the spine called the Atlas, named after the Greek god who supported the heavens. The balancing point of the skull is located slightly behind the centre of gravity, so we have about 40 per cent of our head weight behind the point of balance and 60 per cent in front. We can clearly see that our head would fall forward if it wasn't for the stability provided by our neck muscles.

The free balance of our head on top of the spine can best be seen in young children. A standing child who wishes to walk will subconsciously allow their head to roll forward very slightly on the top of their spine. The weight of their head is effectively put off balance forward and this initiates a lengthening of their back and brings about the correct co-ordination of their muscles to provide the movement. They walk to catch up with their head! The release of our neck is a crucial part of the healthy working of the whole body. As adults, however, we have developed a great many postural habits and one of these is to constantly tighten our neck muscles, pulling our head backward so our face is tilted upward. As this tendency is often accompanied by a stoop or slouch it may not be so obvious.

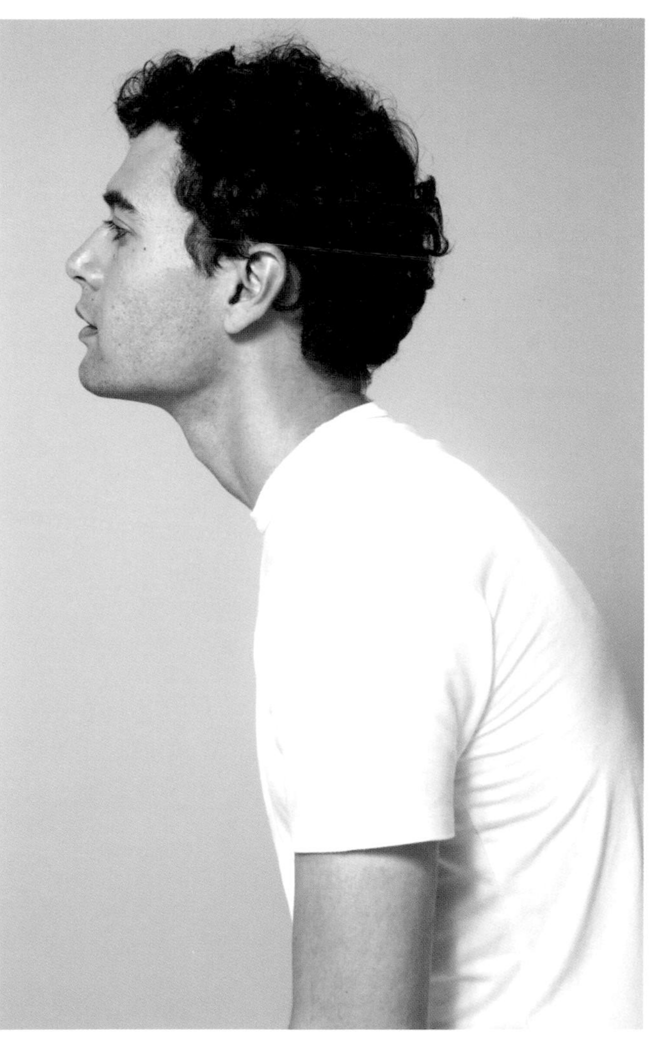

Here the head is held off balance forward of the body causing severe neck tension.

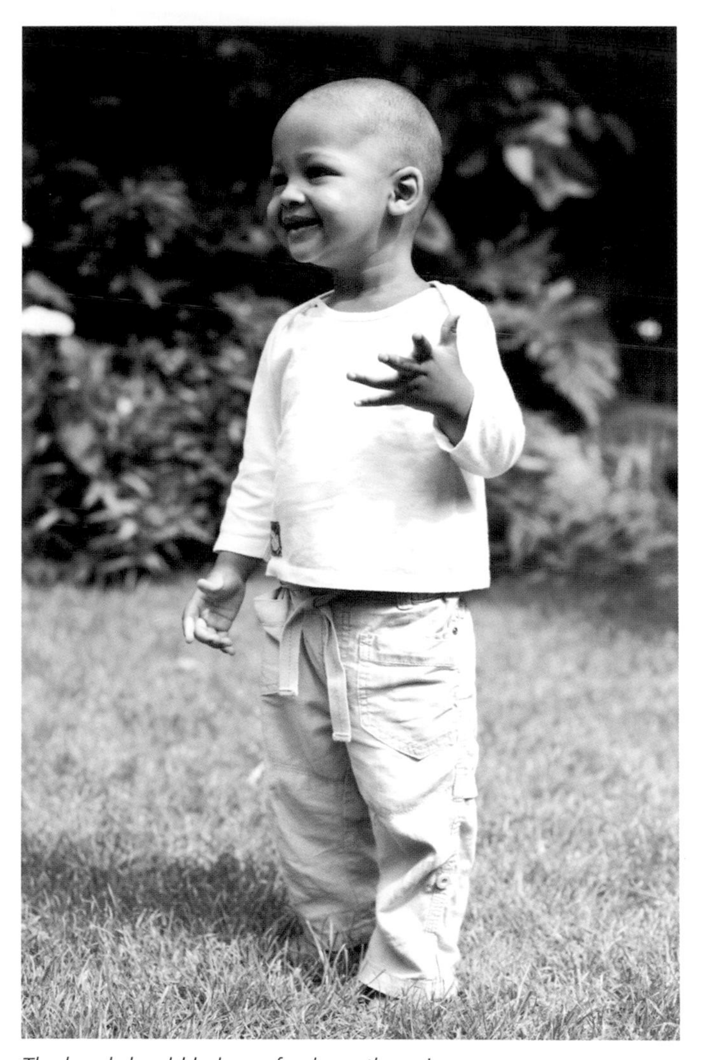

The head should balance freely on the spine.

A lifetime of poor postural habits has resulted in our neck muscles being so strong that we hold our head in rather fixed positions that actively work against free and easy movement. We have a tendency to stiffen our neck and pull our head backward when we want to move forward. We need to allow our head to balance freely in such a way that our neck muscles are not under strain, just like children. We also need to allow our head to roll forward freely as we begin to move so it can initiate a lengthening of our stature as we walk.

The neck is actually formed by the top seven vertebrae of the spine. Many muscles originate here and attach to the bones at the back of the skull; their function is partly to pull the head backward so we look upward, but they also play a role in healthy poise. Given the centre of gravity of the head is in front of the balancing point of the Atlas, these muscles prevent it from falling further forward by acting as a gentle elastic restrainer. However habitual neck tension can smother the subtlety and sensitive working of these muscles so our head no longer balances as it should. Using the Alexander Technique actively encourages these muscles to become more elastic and functional, so our head can balance more freely on top of our spine.

Although our whole neck may be rather stiff, we give significant attention to the top joint where our head balances on the Atlas. We 'direct' our head to balance freely and we do this by thinking. If we truly free our neck a little, it is possible that our head will roll slightly forward on the top joint by its own weight and gravity. It may only nod forward by a millimetre or two, but can be much more if our habitual tendency is to hold our head severely tilted backwards.

To free the neck it is usually helpful to actively allow the head to roll forward by a few millimetres, as this encourages the neck muscles to release some of their contraction; the muscles actually lengthen. Avoid tucking your chin in as this would involve a contraction of muscles in your front. And also avoid letting your head and neck drop forward like a giraffe, as this involves all the vertebrae in your neck and your head will be out of natural alignment. Only allow your head to roll a few millimetres forward on the top vertebra, very high up at a point between your ears. You can think of it as dropping your nose a very small amount.

Freeing the neck is so important to our overall poise and co-ordination that there are extraordinary benefits from persevering with releasing. We may achieve a superficial release fairly quickly, but it is worthwhile sticking with the intention to release the top joint for lengthy periods of not only seconds, but minutes. And when we sense a release, to ask for more, to enquire within and search for more release; to imagine a slight rock of the head forward and even sideways as it 'teeters' on the top of our spine. And when we've released a bit more, we should search again. Do not 'end-gain' by looking for the end result; consider it as an ongoing process.

As your neck becomes freer, the cartilage within the joint may be allowed to expand a bit, providing a springier cushion for your skull to sit on. It may be helpful to think of this cartilage plumping up and supporting your head, lightly and buoyantly. Let it have more space. Enjoy the search for more release. Remember, your head cannot fall off; you are looking for more release than is familiar, so it may feel strange. As you release your neck the arrangement of muscles in your back and the natural springiness of your spine take you upward so you lengthen. Also, the tension-detecting receptors in these sub-occipital muscles can become more sensitive, having been rather smothered by excessive tension in the past. As these receptors regain their sensitivity, our awareness of our head balance and neck tensions can improve.

It is helpful to practise freeing your neck, moment by moment, as often as you can throughout the day. As we move around we will inevitably use our neck muscles, so we need to consciously allow them to be as free as possible all the time. Keeping our neck constantly free is best achieved by constantly freeing it! Release in this area will have a beneficial effect throughout our whole body including our back and legs, right down to our feet.

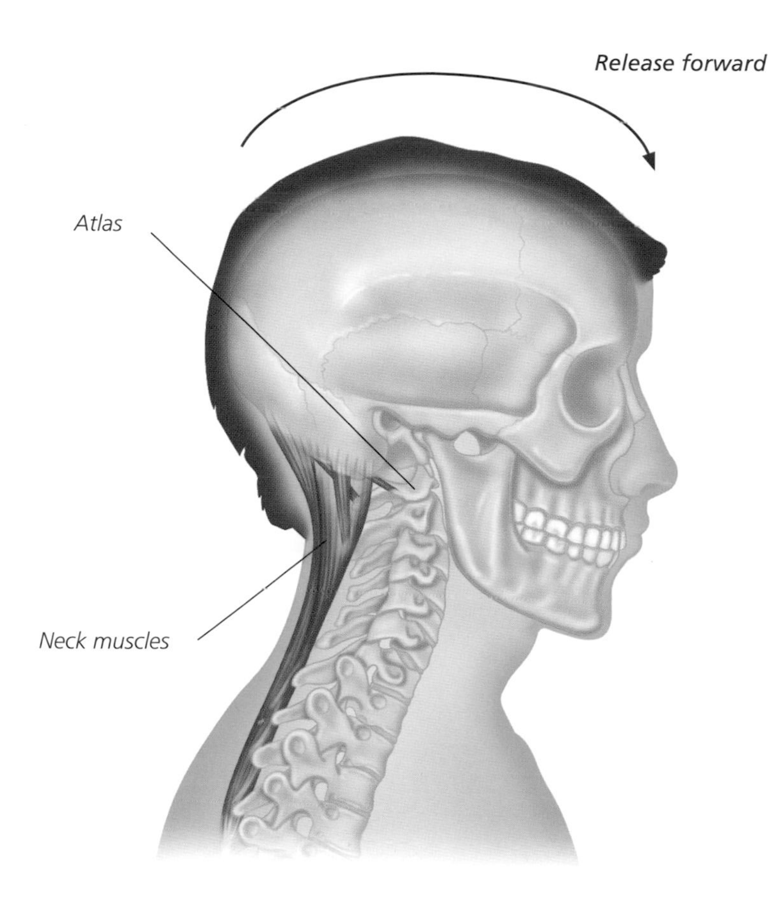

Allow your head to roll forward a few millimetres on the Atlas to help free your neck.

Exercise – Free your neck

›› Be aware of the top of your spine being at a height of roughly between your ears. Allow your head to roll forward just a few degrees on the very top joint, without dropping your neck forward. You might think of your nose dropping a few millimetres. This will help you release your neck. It is not a fixed position but a quality of free poise which is un-held. Think of your head teetering; it should be free like a young child's. Think of the 'cushion' of cartilage supporting your skull plumping up.

Note: Do not tuck your chin in or drop your neck forward. All that is required is release of the muscles at the back of your neck which may result in your head nodding forward slightly.

HELPFUL TIPS

›› Do not try and feel if your neck is stiff or free; the sensitivity of the tension detecting receptors may not be as accurate as you might like, owing to all the tension they have been under for a long time. Don't judge yourself, as you are not sufficiently experienced to know what is right anyway and your sensory perception will be unreliable. Judging yourself only causes frustration. It is far better to adopt a slightly naïve approach and simply follow the guidelines. Stick with the 'means-whereby' approach and let the results look after themselves. As Alexander said, 'You cannot know what is right by an instrument that is wrong.' In short, just think it free.

Information box

The head weighs approximately 4–5kg (9–11lb) and needs to balance freely on the top of the spine at a point roughly between the ears. Forty per cent of the weight of the head is behind the point of balance and 60 per cent of the weight is in front. If we allow our neck muscles to release tension, our head will naturally roll forward a few degrees on the top of our spine, with the help of gravity.

2. Head to go forward and up

Having first freed our neck of tension, we must maintain that quality as we add the intention of our head going forward and upward. Both the freeing of our neck and our intention for our head to go forward and upward bring about a lengthening of our spine.

This second direction is added to the first direction so we simultaneously free the neck and think upward. Directing forward and upward initiates a release of muscle tension and the natural lengthening of our spine and whole stature. It also helps bring about improved muscle co-ordination throughout the whole body. Alexander observed the quality of lengthening in stature in young children and also in vertebrate mammals such as cats, horses and dogs. Any four-legged creature moves forward by first 'sending' its head in a forward direction, lengthening its back and activating its legs to walk. The head is where the eyes, brain and teeth are located and it's the creature's whole intention to get its teeth on what it sees as a potential good lunch. In some respects it is the head that leads and the body's job to carry it around.

Poor postural habits do not allow the natural tendency for the head to lead. A head that is pulled backward with tension is actually going in the wrong direction; it's coming backward and downward when it should be going forward and upward as nature intended.

The line that we want to think of our head travelling in is not vertical, although it is mostly upward. It is actually a few degrees forward of the vertical. Many of us may be habitually dropping our necks forward and down (rather like a giraffe), while also pulling our head backward at the same time. By thinking the first 'direction': 'Let the neck be free', we allow our head to naturally roll forward a few degrees *on the top of the spine* and the second 'direction': 'Allow the head to go forward and up', will bring about a healthier alignment of our neck and back. Note that if your tendency has been to drop your neck forward and down rather like a giraffe, then directing your head upward (by thinking) will encourage your neck to come back, so your head weight is more over your shoulders.

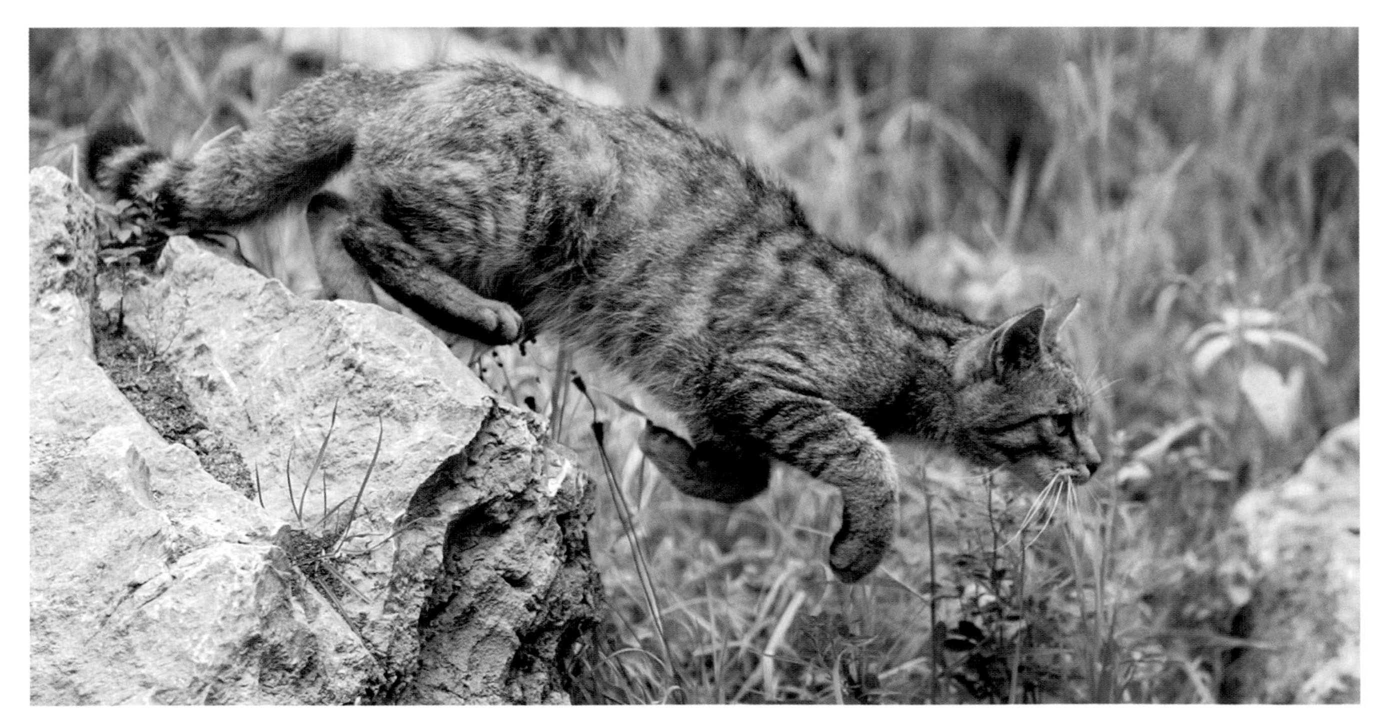

A cat sends its head forward as it springs. The head leads and the body follows.

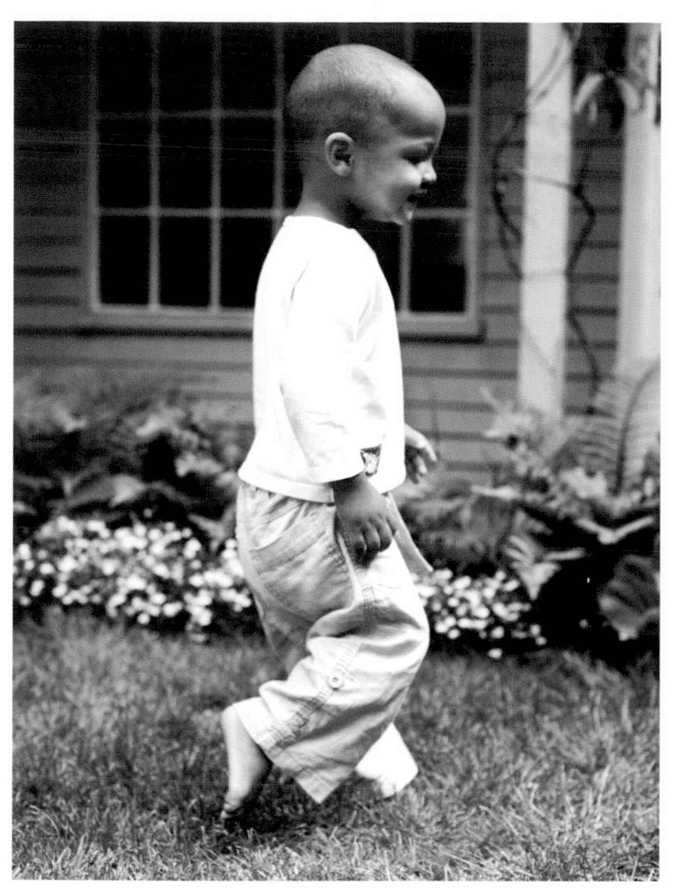

Child lengthening as he walks.

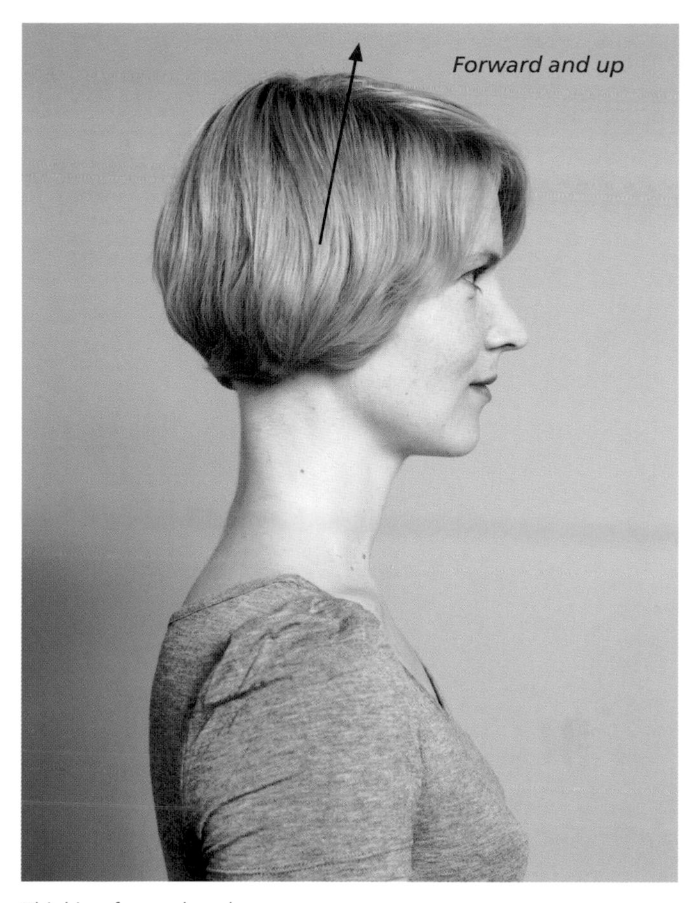

Thinking forward and up.

Exercise – Allow your head to go forward and up

›› First 'direct' your neck to be free (particularly on the Atlas vertebra) so your head teeters on top of your spine. While maintaining the freedom of your neck, think and send your head in a forward and upward direction. Do not push or make any effort whatsoever as this will cause tension. You need to release unwanted tension (not make more tension!) and then 'direct' your head in a forward and upward direction. This realigns your neck and initiates the lengthening and support of your entire back.

HELPFUL TIPS

›› When directing your head forward and upward, become interested in the air space above your head. Where you put your attention is where you are drawn towards. Think of the air space above you and imagine your head can go up into it. But ensure you do not make any physical effort.

3. Back to lengthen

The next step in the sequence of directions involves keeping the first two in mind while adding the third of lengthening in our back. While freeing our neck we add, 'Head to go forward and up', and then, 'Back to lengthen'. These directions are thought, one after each other, all together.

We wish our back to lengthen from the bottom to the top. So, if we are sitting, the bottom of our back would be the sitting bones under our pelvis that are in contact with the chair and we lengthen right up to the crown of our head. This 'direction' does not only mean 'lengthen the spine', but the whole area of our back. When standing we 'lengthen' from our heels to the crown of our head.

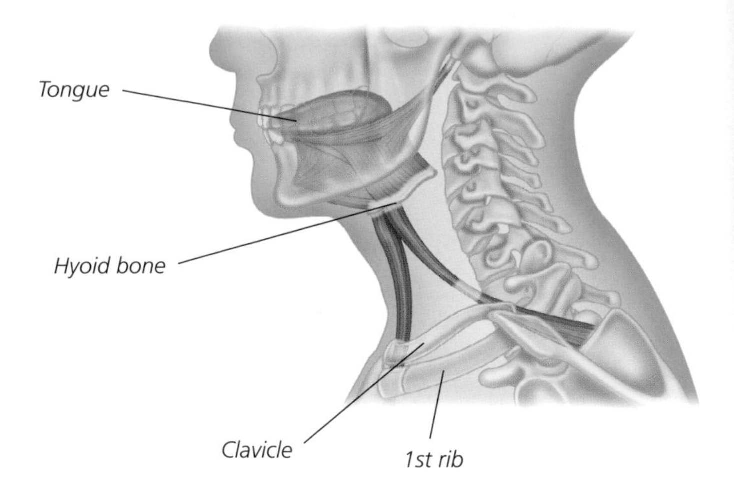

With postural habits, it is very common for shortening to occur in the back in a variety of ways. A shortening of stature can be the result of slouching so the lumbar spine collapses squashing the tummy, or an over-arching and hollowing of the back that can squash the lumbar discs (lordosis), an excessive rounding of the upper back (kyphosis), a sideways twist in the back (scoliosis), or a combination of these conditions. All these versions of shortening in stature put the back under enormous strain, causing excessive tension, compression of the inter-vertebral discs as well as pressing on nerves. They also cause a reduction of internal capacity for the internal organs which can affect their healthy functioning.

Giving the 'direction' to lengthen involves thinking, wishing or visualising; it is a clear mental intention for this to happen. It is quite likely that we will not feel anything happening at the precise moment that we think it, but we should 'inhibit' making any effort as it will hamper the change to our co-ordination. We should give the 'order' to lengthen then *allow* it. A change in the co-ordination of all our muscles will reduce the excessive effort that some muscles are habitually making while engaging other muscles to support us in the manner they should. Any twists or excessive curvature that we have experienced in the past is the result of inefficient use of muscle and will be improved by our new co-ordination.

However, while directing our back to lengthen, we must also not forget the front of our body which can be in quite a shortened condition. If we do not allow our front to lengthen too, then we will bow over like a banana. The lengthening that we would like applies to the whole body. A great many ailments to do with digestion, bowel movements, breathing and circulation are caused by our chronic tendency to shorten the distance from the groin to our throat. If we are shortening in front, we effectively compress and reduce the internal capacity of our thorax so all our organs are squashed. Shortening in the front of our body is caused by lack of awareness of our condition during the many activities we do throughout our day, such as sitting at a desk, riding a bicycle. It's my view that shortening in our front is one of the greatest ills of modern mankind. However it cannot be addressed in isolation as our body works as a unified whole; there are compensations throughout our whole body.

As we think, 'Back to lengthen', let us also remember that we wish to lengthen in our front too, from the groin to our throat. Think 'up' in front as well as in our back. But beware of trying to lengthen in front at the expense of lengthening in your back as you will begin to arch and shorten your back. Remember it is a thinking method, not a doing method.

Exercise – Allow your back to lengthen

›› First 'direct' your neck to be free in the manner described previously. While keeping that going, think of your head going in a forward and upward direction. When you are managing to maintain a free neck and think upward with your head, add the idea of your back lengthening. It is most important that you 'inhibit' any tendency to make a physical effort as this will cause muscle contraction and shortening. You must *think* your directions. Do not worry about the end result.

›› Think: 'Neck to be free, head to go forward and up, back to lengthen.'

›› Give the orders and allow it to happen.

Tip

›› Release the tongue so it lies flat with the tip behind your lower teeth. Allow the hyoid bone and the collarbones to come up as you release the muscles in the front of your throat. These releases will allow more overall lengthening in front.

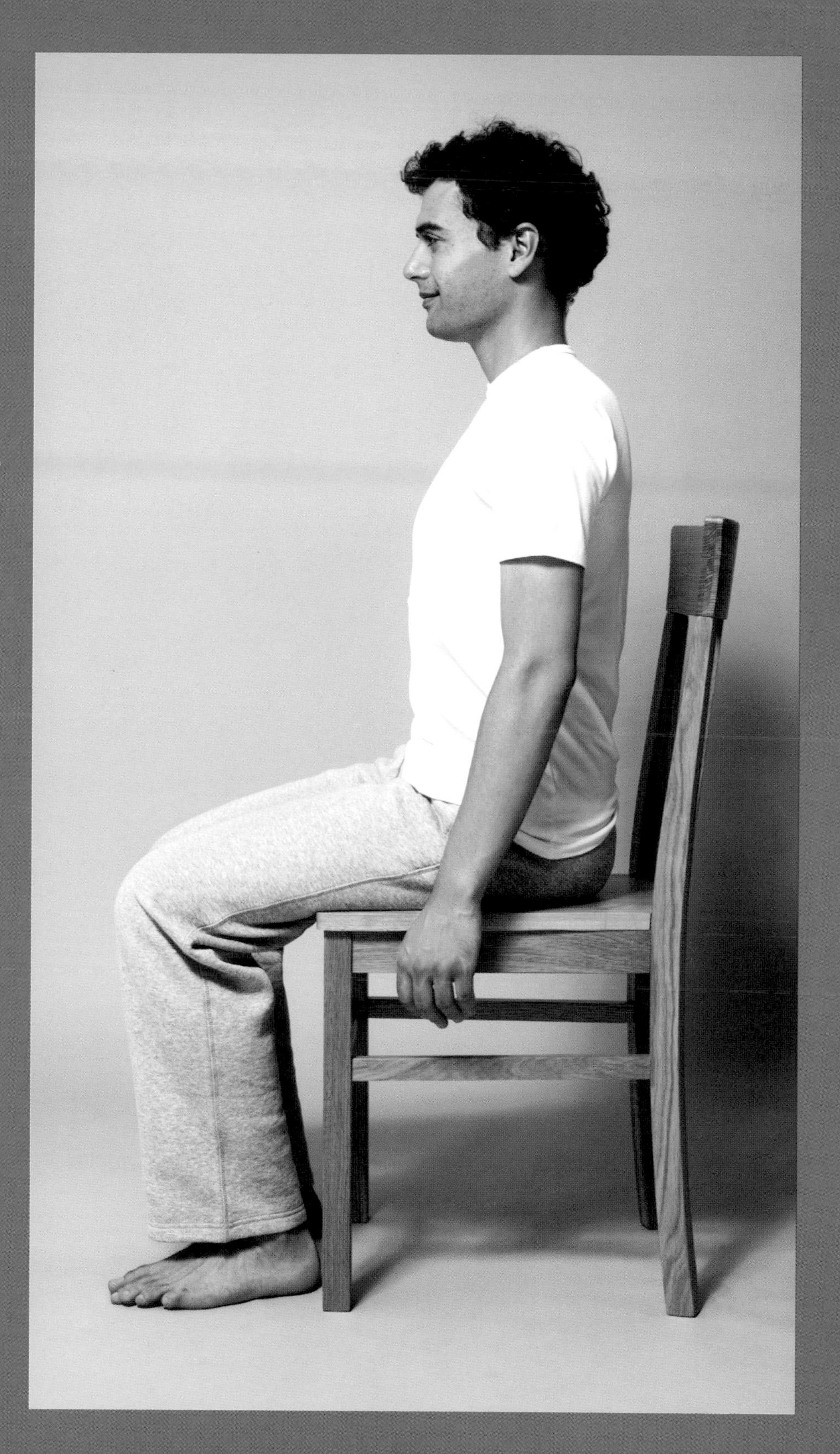

4. Back to widen

The next step in the sequence of directions involves keeping the first three directions in mind while adding the fourth direction of our back to widen. Allowing our back to widen means giving the freedom to the whole of our torso to open out and broaden. Our size or shape may not alter by thinking this direction, but giving the mental 'order' will help to encourage an improvement of the co-ordination of muscles throughout our whole body as well as providing the maximum internal capacity of our thorax.

The efficient working of our body does not involve having relaxed muscles; far from it. Our muscles exist in order to work, to support us and move us around. However, a lifetime of habitual narrowing brings about problems such as an over-arched back, pinching between our shoulder blades, rounded shoulders, hollowed chest, tightly held ribs and inefficient breathing.

The direction to widen applies to various parts of the torso, not only the back. For instance, if we give the direction to widen across the middle of the back, we must 'inhibit' any tendency to narrow in the front by pulling the shoulders forward or hollowing the chest. The whole of the torso should 'widen' to bring about the correct co-ordination of muscles.

We think of widening:

1. **Across the lumbar back.**
2. **Across the middle thoracic back.**
3. **Across our upper thoracic back between our shoulder blades.**

When you have become accustomed to the main directions, you should practise thinking of the widening of each of the following areas to bring about maximum expansiveness. Be sure to use no effort.

Think of widening:

4. **Across the front of the chest from your chest bone out to the shoulders.**
5. **Widen within both armpits so each hollow is more open.**
6. **Between the armpits; away from one another.**
7. **Across the top of the shoulders.**

By working out in a gym we can make various muscles in our back stronger, but this does not mean that these muscles will work together in a naturally co-ordinated way to support us without a sense of effort when we are walking, sitting or bending. It's not so much the individual strength of muscles that's important, but how we use what we've got. When we encourage lengthening and widening of our back, our muscles become very supportive and strong, like a trampoline. A strong back is a widening back.

The directions we give to widen our torso may not change our physical size or shape, but if we have been particularly narrowing or shortening then we will help ourselves re-establish our full stature. But this is not our primary consideration. We give our directions because they will organise our muscles to work together in better co-ordination and our shape may change as a consequence of this.

We are effectively spring-loaded. The conscious attitude (or subconscious as it is in children and animals) to be expansive releases tensions that pull us downward and inward, and the natural springiness of our spine and ribs will allow us to extend upward and outward. This activates our 'anti-gravity' mechanism in response to the Earth's gravitational pull, bringing about better co-ordination and strength. This is how it is in nature.

[Note: The directions to lengthen and widen should not be applied independently. They are part of a sequence that is self regulating so we do not over-lengthen or over-widen. Apply them one after the other.]

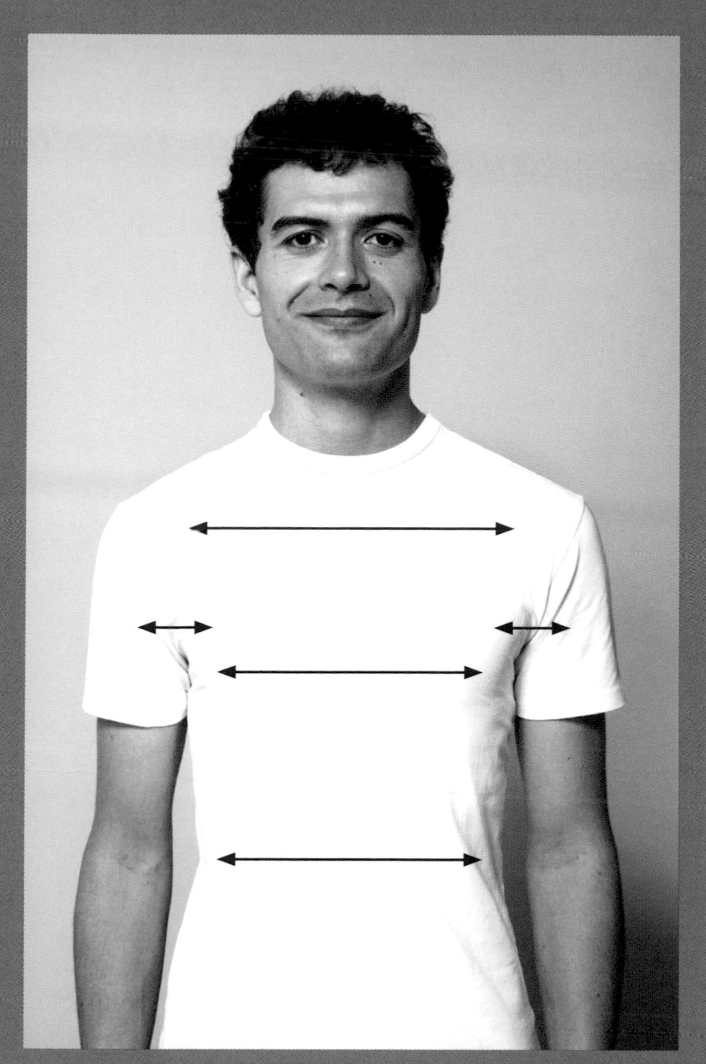
Think of widening across your front...

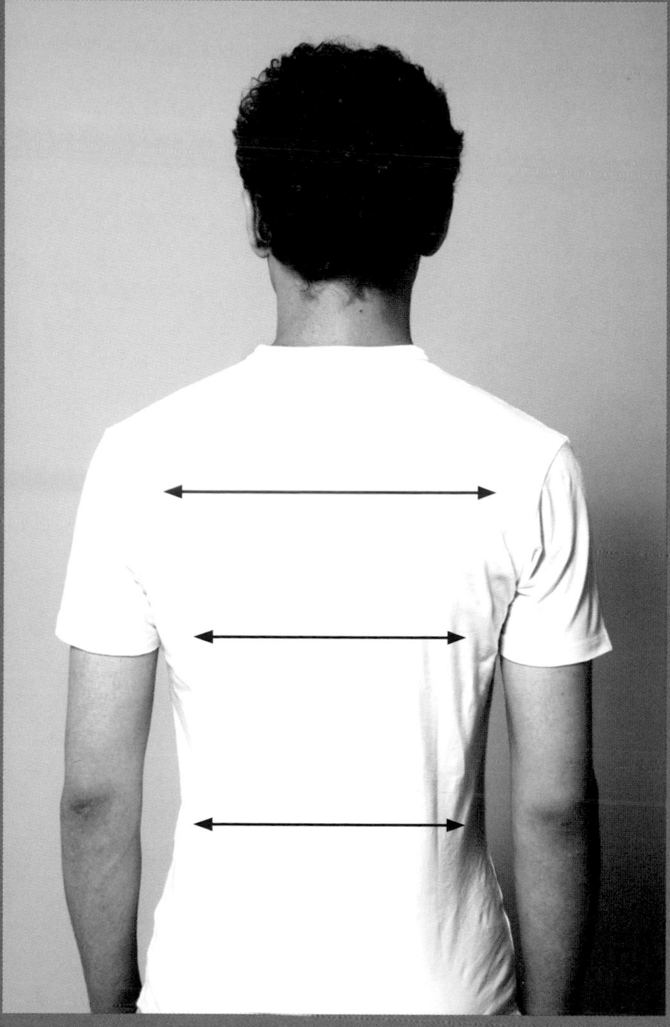
...and widening across your back.

Exercise – Allow your back to widen

›› It is essential that you start the sequence of 'direction' from the beginning in the correct order. First 'direct' your neck to be free in the manner described previously. Second add 'head to go forward and upward'. Third, add 'back to lengthen'. Fourth, 'direct' your 'back to widen'. Again, it is most important that you 'inhibit' any tendency to make a physical effort as this will cause a shortening and narrowing of your stature. You must 'think' your directions.

›› Think: 'Neck to be free, head to go forward and upward, back to lengthen and widen.'

›› Think each 'direction' for a few moments before adding the next 'direction'. We should think these directions, one after each other, all together.

5. Knees to go forward and away

When we have given all the other main directions in the sequence given, we should 'direct' our knees to go forward and away.

A common problem is the contraction of the muscles in the upper legs which draws the knees toward the pelvis. This tendency causes unnecessary tension in the lower back possibly resulting in stiffness and a hollowing and narrowing of the back as well as tension within the hip and groin area.

The 'direction' 'Allow knees to go forward and away' works in conjunction with the other directions, which should be given first in the correct order. Allowing the knees to go forward and away applies when sitting, standing or walking. It can be more easily understood if we first consider sitting. When sitting upright so our weight goes down through our sitting bones into the chair, our feet should be flat on the floor and spaced out slightly wider than our hips. Our feet should not be turned inward or outward, but should be in line with our legs. Now we should 'direct' our knees to go forward, away from our pelvis. We might like to think of our knees 'going' to the far-away wall in the room. However they also need to be directed slightly away from each other, first because our legs are angled outward, and second to inhibit the tendency to draw the knees toward each other which causes tensions down the inside of the leg and in the groin. Our knees should be directed in a line over the big toes. By 'thinking' our knees to go forward and away, we help release many muscles of the upper legs that attach to either side of the lumbar spine and which can cause the back to tense and hollow if they over-contract. A common cause of a tight back is our tendency to tighten and shorten the inside of our legs. This 'direction' works along with all the other directions and can really help avoid back pain.

Directing our knees to go forward and away encourages the proper action of our legs when we stand up from a sitting position or bend to sit down. It is a question of allowing our knees to go forward and away, which is actually what they will do if we cease to tense and pull them backward and inward. These directions are preventative orders; to prevent the wrong thing from happening.

When walking, knees should be directed forward and away to help release the lower back and aid the correct action of the legs. This will be discussed in detail in Chapter 5.

We can give all five principal directions, one after the other. Think each 'direction' for a few moments, before adding the next 'direction', then repeat again. These directions are not a mantra. Each 'direction' requires us to 'intend' it to happen. We must 'mean' it and allow it. Do not repeat the directions over and over again while thinking about something else. By bringing our full attention to them, we will enable our directions to have the strongest influence on our co-ordination and poise.

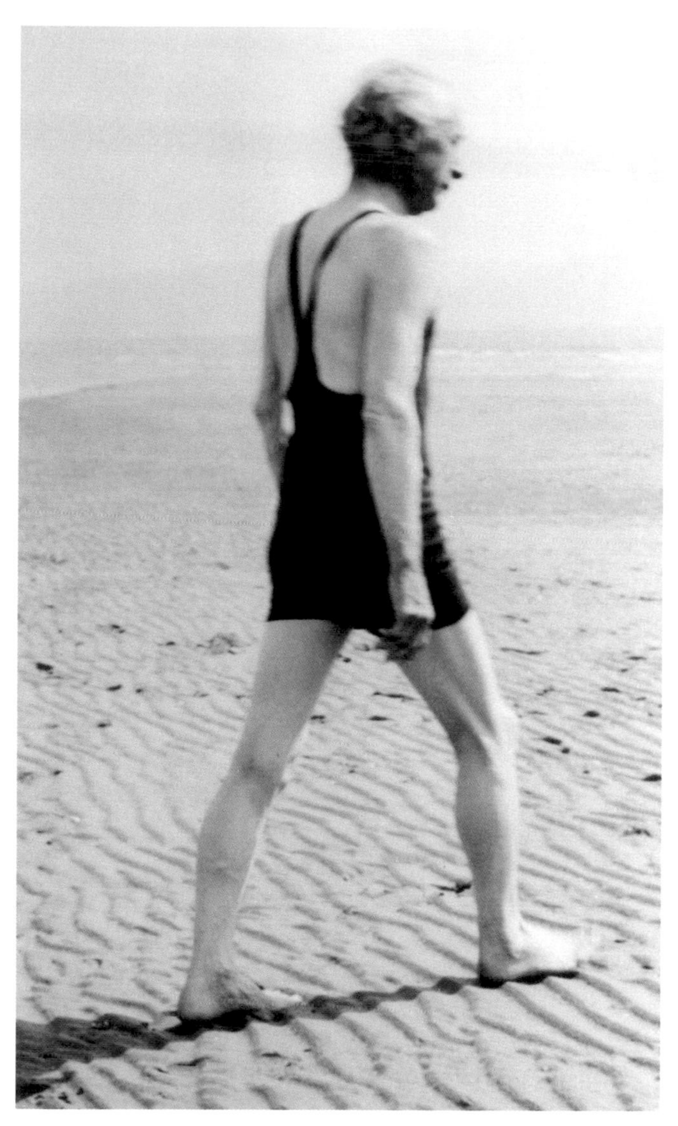

F.M. Alexander lengthening in stature and sending his knees forward and away, while walking along a beach.

Exercise – Allow your knees to go forward and away

›› Start by giving the sequence of directions from the beginning in the correct order described above. 'Direct' your neck to be free; second, 'send' your head forward and upward. Third, 'direct' your back to lengthen then 'direct' your back to widen. Once you have clearly thought these four directions, add the fifth 'direction': 'Knees to go forward and away'. Again, it is most important that you 'inhibit' any tendency to make a physical effort. It is more a question of releasing them to go forward and away, which is actually what they will do if we cease to tense and pull them backward and inward. You must 'think' your directions.

›› Think: 'Neck to be free, head to go forward and upward, back to lengthen and widen, knees to go forward and away.' Think each 'direction' for a few moments before adding the next one. We should think these directions, one after the other, all together.

Primary Control

In Alexander's third book *The Use of the Self* he stated:

> There is a primary control of the use of the self which governs the working of all the mechanisms and so renders the control of the complex human organism comparatively simple.

He discovered that the healthy working of the whole body is governed to a high degree by the relationship of the head, neck and back. When this relationship is upset, it has a detrimental effect on our whole co-ordination, balance and ease of movement. In the healthy movement of all mammals, the head leads the way for the spine to lengthen, allowing the limbs to move freely in relation to the back, so the entire creature moves as a co-ordinated whole.

These parts must not be held fixed; it is their interrelationship that governs the correct working of our whole body, including arms and legs. If this relationship is disturbed, our overall co-ordination is upset. We should consider our neck as a continuation of our back, with gentle curvature of our spine continuing right up to under our skull. Our head needs to balance freely on the top vertebra of our spine.

By giving directions for our head to go forward and up, we enable the musculature to support us with the appropriate combination of length and curve to our spine in a supple and elastic way. So, without dropping our neck forward, we should allow our head to 'tend' forward on the top vertebra called the Atlas, allowing our back to come backward into more vertical alignment which in turn enables it to lengthen. We need to maintain good Primary Control of our 'use' in order to promote muscular harmony throughout the body, because the head-neck-back relationship dominates the partial pattern of the limbs. The healthy and pain-free working of our arms, wrists and hands, such as when playing an instrument will be aided by maintaining good Primary Control. We achieve good Primary Control by applying the principal directions that we discussed earlier in this chapter: 'Allow the neck to be free, head to go forward and upward, back to lengthen and widen, and knees to go forward and away.' During our daily activities, we should try to remember these directions. We should pause and 'inhibit', to give ourselves time to think, then we can go through the directions. By 'inhibiting' first, then applying the thoughtful directions, we maintain good Primary Control.

It should be noted, when we have given our directions in such a way as to encourage the correct co-ordination of our musculature, it may feel wrong, but gradually, as our sensory perception improves, it will feel more right. What we will feel as being right is not the posture or position, but the correct 'direction'.

> There is no such thing as a right position, but there is such a thing as a right direction.
>
> F. M. Alexander

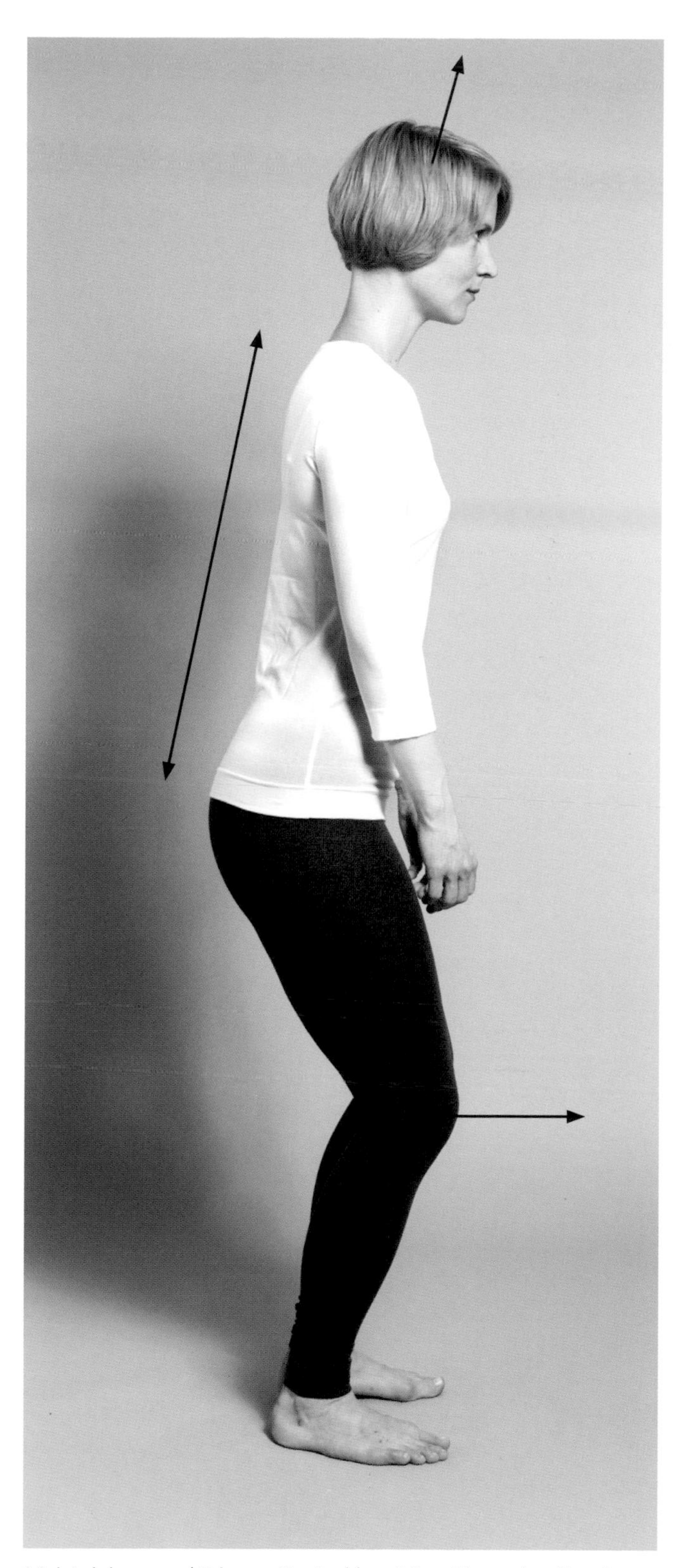

Maintaining good Primary Control by giving Alexander directions.

Once we have achieved some improvement to our poise and sense of well-being, we should not hold onto what we feel as that would cause fixation and stiffness. To maintain what we are experiencing and to improve further, we should cast it aside and re-apply the directions that brought about our improvement in the first place. What we actually want can only be achieved in the process of looking for it. I shall repeat that again as it is so important: the quality of free and expansive poise we want can only be experienced by the process of looking for it, because as soon as we try to hold onto it, we have lost the very quality we want.

Life is about living one moment after the other. We should 'give our directions' again and again as we bend, walk, sit or run. We need to maintain a constant condition of free expansiveness, moment after moment, even if we are simply sitting. The philosopher John Dewey called it 'thinking in activity'. By giving our directions in this way – i.e. by constantly freeing our neck, sending our head forward and upward, by directing our back to lengthen and widen and our knees to go forward and away – we are maintaining good primary control over the use of ourselves.

HELPFUL TIPS

›› When we feel that we have made some improvement to our poise, we must not hold onto the feeling or the position as this will cause fixation and stiffness. To maintain what we are experiencing and to improve further, we should cast aside what we feel we have gained and re-apply the directions that brought about our improvements in the first place. What we actually want can only be had in the process of looking for it. Forget the end result, work on the process.

Awareness of space

As adults we probably have very little awareness of space around us compared to how we were as children. Toddlers 'own' the space around them; they are gregarious, outgoing, expansive in nature and stature. Our perception of ourselves tends to be restricted to the body we can touch but little awareness of the space we take up. It is helpful to be aware of the space immediately above our head that we could 'move into' as we think of 'lengthening' and the space around us as we 'widen'. By thinking expansively we can 'fill the room' and benefit hugely as our physique responds to the expansive thought.

We also have space within us which can easily be reduced by postural and tensional habits. The Alexander Technique helps us eliminate these tendencies and encourage natural expansiveness. Our body will work more efficiently and suffer from less discomfort if we help ourselves be expansive. Our spine is more flexible if it's lengthening; our joints will be more supple with less wear and tear if they are allowed to expand by lengthening and widening; and our organs will function better if our vital capacity is as large as possible.

By Directing we are mentally instructing one part of us away from another, to lengthen and widen. Indeed it is possible to Direct any part of us away from another and achieve release of tension. You can direct your fingers to lengthen, the space between your fingers to widen which will help release your wrists and hands. Direct your armpits to open out and to go away from one another to open out your chest. Or direct your hip joints to widen away from each other to release your hips.

But it must be remembered that individual thoughts of Direction and expansiveness are secondary to applying the Primary Control. Fragmented thinking won't work. It's got to be seen and used as part of the overall guiding instructions. So, give your Directions in the sequence described on page 73 and do be aware of the space around you that you wish to move into. Think 'out of the box'. Think beyond your body to the space around you that you could expand into; this may be a few millimetres or up to the ceiling or the sky and horizon. Think expansively and you'll trigger a positive physical response.

Tips

›› Be aware of the space above your head that you can move into. Direct your head up into that space.

›› Be aware of the space around you that you can expand into. Direct to widen into the space on either side of you.

Core strength

It is a commonly held belief that if we have backache or wish to avoid it, we need to build core strength in order to support the spine. Core-strengthening programmes involve strengthening certain trunk muscles that may be under-used as well as the ligaments and muscles surrounding the spine. If we play contact sports and need to hold off opponents this will be very helpful, however it should not be necessary in our normal life of moving around, standing, sitting and bending.

The supportive muscles of our trunk and around our spine can become under-used by habits such as slouching, and a degree of muscle tone is required to support our tummy and contain the gut. But there are some issues with building core strength as a means of rectifying a back problem. First, the exercising and strengthening of muscles does not mean that they will work together in a co-ordinated way to support us in daily life. Strength does not equal co-ordination and support. Second, we do not see toddlers with lots of core strength and they have wonderful upright poise and are well co-ordinated. As children we have very soft tummy and trunk muscles yet we stand and sit very freely and at our full height.

Building core strength to rectify a bad back does not address the actual cause of the problem as it only compensates for the lack of co-ordination throughout our musculature. What we are actually lacking is 'direction', the sort of 'direction' we can see in young children as well as our companion vertebrates such as cats and horses, as we have previously discussed. A lack of 'direction' causes our torso to collapse, so we end up slouched with back pain. Strengthening our core muscles around an inactive back will bring about support, rather like a corset, but it won't necessarily encourage the lengthening and widening required for good co-ordination. It may take the pressure off the discs, but the resulting tension is more than likely to cause a shortening of stature and reduction of vital capacity.

We can only achieve our full expansiveness if our muscles are 'commanded' to work in the manner for which they were designed. As in the case of four-legged creatures where their head leads the way forward, our muscles are activated to bring about upright tall stature without any sense of effort if we have the inner intention to be tall. We too need to lead the way with our head but we do so upward as we are bipeds on two feet. It is not effort or strength that is required to support a weak back, but better muscle co-ordination. Applying the directions in the Alexander Technique brings about healthy use of our musculature and as the muscles begin to work to support us in the way they should, they will support our back and become stronger to do the job required of them. But they will become stronger, not by the isolation of muscles and by individual strengthening, but by all working together for the purpose they were intended: to support us in movement, sitting and standing. They will also allow greater flexibility and suppleness so we can bend and twist more easily.

Gym work and strengthening exercises can cause excessive tensions to build up which can work against good co-ordination. Walking, running and aerobic exercise will bring cardio-vascular benefits while still enabling expansive use of the body. The lifting of weights can be quite detrimental to back problems and should really only be attempted once your co-ordination is adequately refined so you remain in good balance in a free and lengthening stature. One of the dangers of gym work-outs is the distraction of videos and loud music that allow us to do repetitive gym work without care and attention to how we are doing it. Alexander Technique lessons and the guidelines in this book will help provide you with the co-ordination and good use necessary to avoid strain when exercising.

More about releasing unwanted tensions

As we discussed earlier, backache is not a condition that solely relates to our back; if the cause is postural, the use of the whole body is involved. Improving our poise to enable it to function healthily and without backache requires the inhibition of harmful tensional habits as well as giving of directions. 'Inhibiting' harmful habits involves bringing our awareness to our situation in any activity, even when just sitting on a chair or standing. Let us now look at some additional ways in which we can help ourselves.

Using your eyes to free your neck

How you use your eyes affects your neck. It might be surprising at first to consider that our eyes might contribute to neck tension, but a change in the manner in which we look around can help our neck and back become freer.

To enable you to move your head freely and without unnecessary tension, look with your eyes in that direction first. Simplistic? Let's consider this in more detail.

Many of us suffer from neck tension, stiffness and reduced mobility and it is often the case that when we look over our shoulder, or even to the left or right, we use more tension than necessary; we may also pull our head backward with excessive muscle contraction and even close our eyes. And if we have difficulty in turning our head we resort to turning our whole body, rather than moving our eyes, yet the eyes are actually designed to move in any direction. Just watch a two-year-old looking around; they always turn their eyes before they turn their head.

There are six muscles attached to each eye to make them move up, down and sideways, plus another muscle connected to the upper eyelid so this moves automatically when we look up. The nerves from these muscles pass through our head, passing between some of the neck muscles to enter the spinal cord, on their way to the brain. Interestingly, if we have a habit of stiffening our neck, which most of us do, this puts pressure on the nerves to our eyes (as well as other parts of the body), so they have a stiffening effect on our eye mobility. By freeing our neck from tension we can positively affect the functioning of our eyes but also, in addition, if we encourage more eye movement, this helps the freedom in our neck.

Exercise – Moving your eyes

›› Sit reasonably upright in a chair and experiment to see if your eye movement can help the mobility of your neck. The objective is to use minimal effort during the movement.

›› First give some time to freeing your neck. Allow your head to balance 'freely' on top of your spine at a point roughly between your ears. Think of your head 'teetering'. To help you release your neck, allow your head to roll forward just a few degrees, i.e. let your nose drop a few millimetres and look out straight ahead of you. Refer to page 74. Direct your head forward and upwards, back to lengthen.

›› You are now going to turn your head to the left, but do not turn immediately; look with your eyes to the tip of your left shoulder but *do not turn your head.* If you can't quite see your shoulder, just look in that general direction. Now simply *allow* your head to turn to follow your eyes. Do not actively turn your head at all, but simply give permission for your head to follow your eyes. It's so easy to use far more effort than required. Think of it being so free your head can just 'float' round. To return, look with your eyes straight ahead and simply give your head permission to follow. If this was not your experience, then try again. Now do the same exercise to the right. Look first at the tip of your right shoulder, then just allow your head to follow. Think of it floating round. Was this any easier than you normally experience? You might like to practise this periodically to help your neck tension and overall co-ordination.

›› If you're going to look somewhere or turn in a particular direction, it's very helpful to look with your eyes in that direction first. It seems simplistic, but it can be most helpful.

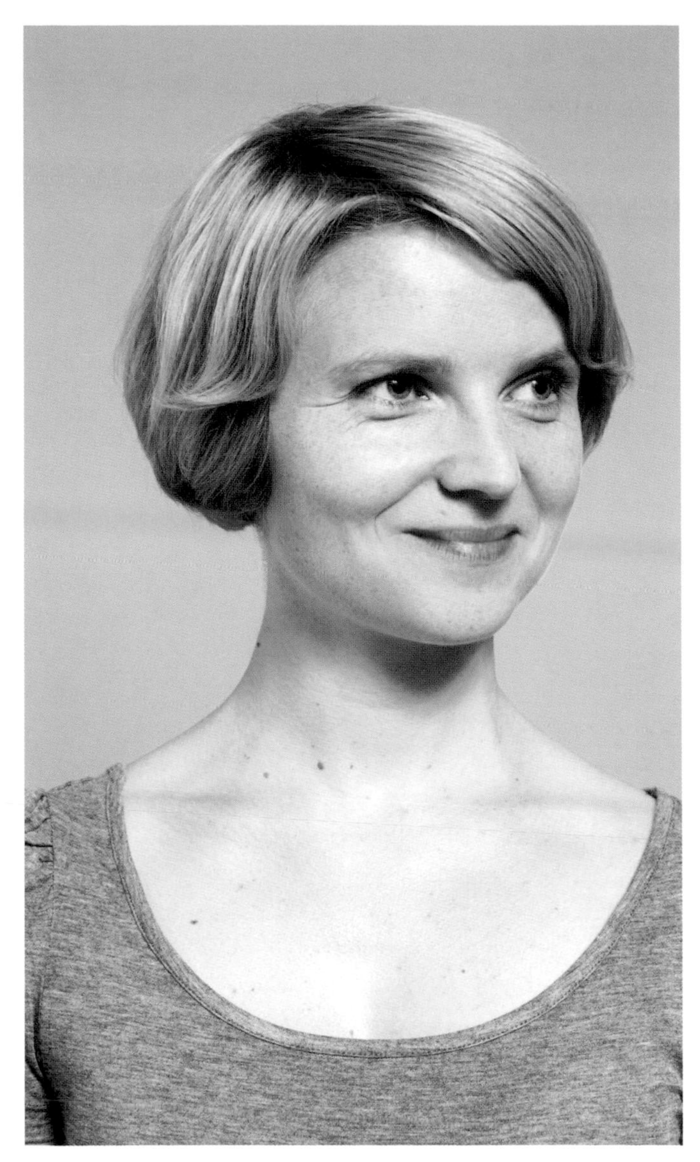

Move your eyes when looking around to help free your neck.

The use of our eyes is linked closely with the movement of our body, understandable when we consider that one main function of our eyes is to see where we're going! There is a strong connection between hand and eye; move one and the other will follow in that direction more easily than otherwise.

Releasing your shoulders

Shoulders can be very prone to habitual tension as they are linked closely to our 'fight or flight' reflex. They are a very complex arrangement of muscle, ligaments and bones so there are an infinite number of ways we may 'interfere' by pulling them out of natural alignment. We should take care how we redress the situation.

It would be very easy, with our 'end-gaining' habits, to try to adjust our shoulders so they appear 'correct'. If our shoulders are pulled forward, we may feel that they should be pulled back. But this approach is just fidgeting with the situation and can only lead to further problems. If our shoulders, for example, are pulled or rounded forward, it is because we are actually causing it to happen with muscle tensions. It would be a mistake to try and pull them back as this would involve tensing muscles between our shoulder blades; the end result would be further tension created to counteract the tension that is pulling them out of alignment, creating a royal battle of tensions that would cause more stiffness and rigidity. Our shoulders would enjoy a natural and healthy alignment if we ceased pulling them forward in the first place! Our approach should be to inhibit our habits of tensing in this harmful way so they become free of tension, broad and expansive, with no strain in our neck.

The same approach applies if our shoulders are hunched up around our ears, or drooping down, or narrowed by constantly pulling them backward.

There is no correct position as such for us to 'hold' our shoulders, as the holding would cause tension and fixation. The answer is to release them to let them find their own natural alignment. However, we can give them a 'correct' direction. If we 'direct' our shoulders to be free and wide, but avoid any attempt to adjust them, then the direction (thought instruction) will bring about a natural change in our muscle co-ordination.

Shoulders are not separate from our back but are an integral part of our torso. Considering the large flat sheet muscles of the trapezius in our upper back and latissimus dorsi that spans the back and connects to our upper arm, we can clearly see how releasing shoulder tension is an important aspect of helping us avoid back pain.

Remember, healthy natural poise does not require effort; we just need to 'leave ourselves alone' and give ourselves the correct direction.

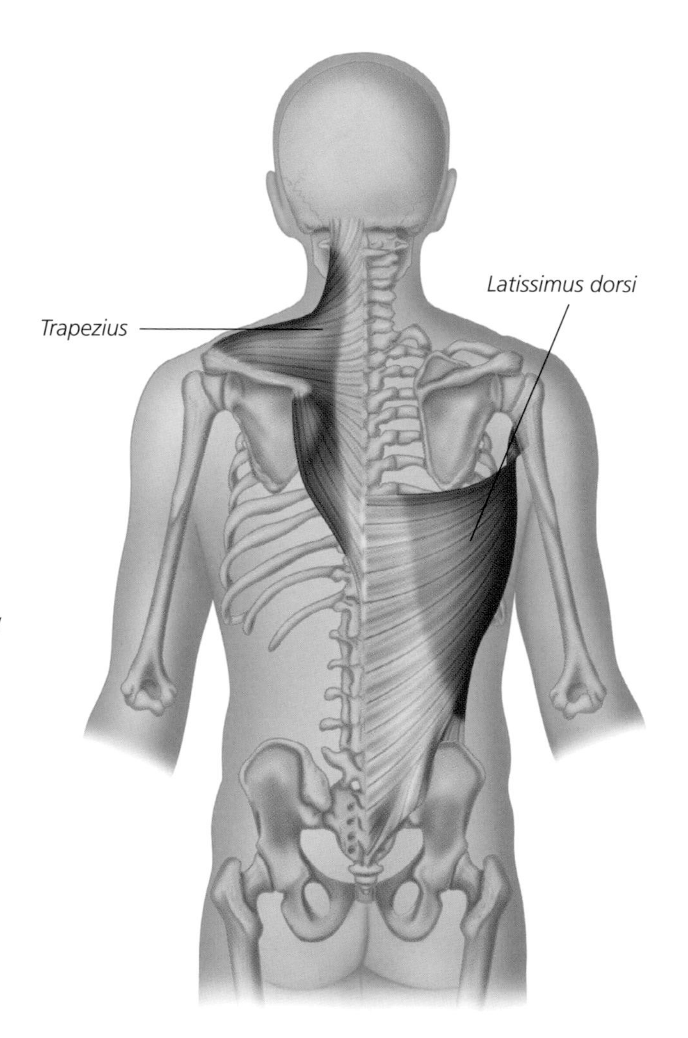

The Trapezius and Latissimus Dorsi muscles span across your back.

Releasing tension in the hips and legs

When our back is not working well it is likely that the upper back, shoulders and hips will also be affected. With a weak back, for instance, our hip and leg muscles can be forced to work overtime as many of the leg muscles extend right up into our pelvis and lower back.

Releasing our hips and legs when standing, sitting or walking relies on the improvement of our whole muscular co-ordination. We need the free balance of our head on our neck and our 'intention' for our head to go forward and upward, our back to lengthen and widen, and our knees to go forward and away. These directions will bring about healthy co-ordination of the whole body including our hips and legs.

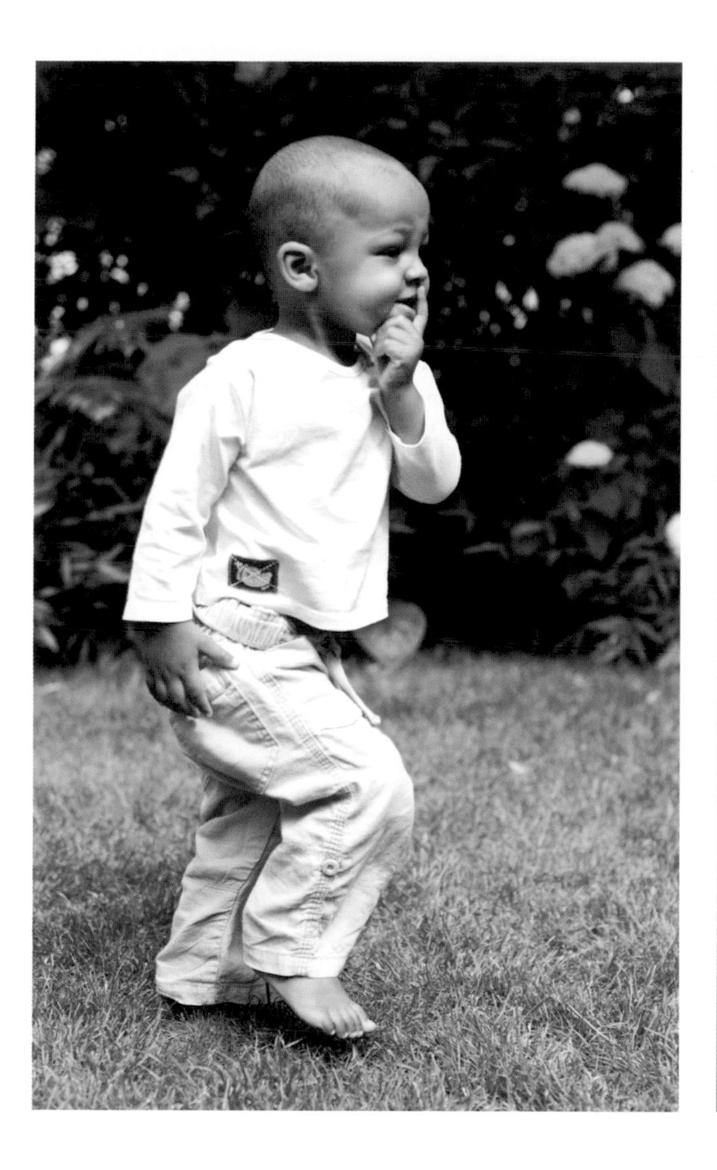

Exercise – Walking with knees going forward and away

›› When walking, actively point your knees in the direction you are walking, so they go forward and away, over the big toe of each foot. First free your neck and 'direct' your head upward, back to lengthen and widen, then send each knee forward and slightly away from each other. You may feel that you are picking up your feet more and this will help you avoid leaning forward when walking. Endeavour to walk with the minimum of effort; your legs should release out of each hip with every step. Let your legs move freely.

Releasing tension in the hands and wrists

The idea of releasing our hands and wrists may seem only appropriate if we suffer from Repetitive Strain Injury (RSI) but as with any other part of us they relate to our whole poise. Tension in our thumbs is linked closely to tight armpits and hunched shoulders, which in turn affect the proper engagement and co-ordination of our back muscles. Releasing our thumbs and wrists can be an important aid in helping our back to function healthily.

It is a good principle to allow your hands and wrists to relax as much and as often as possible. We tend to over-use the muscles in our forearms and hands as a matter of habit, and even those of us who do not have RSI may well suffer the consequences. So when typing, ensure your forearms are horizontal to your wrists or slightly higher and use as little effort as possible in your fingers. Also, think broad across your shoulders and between your armpits.

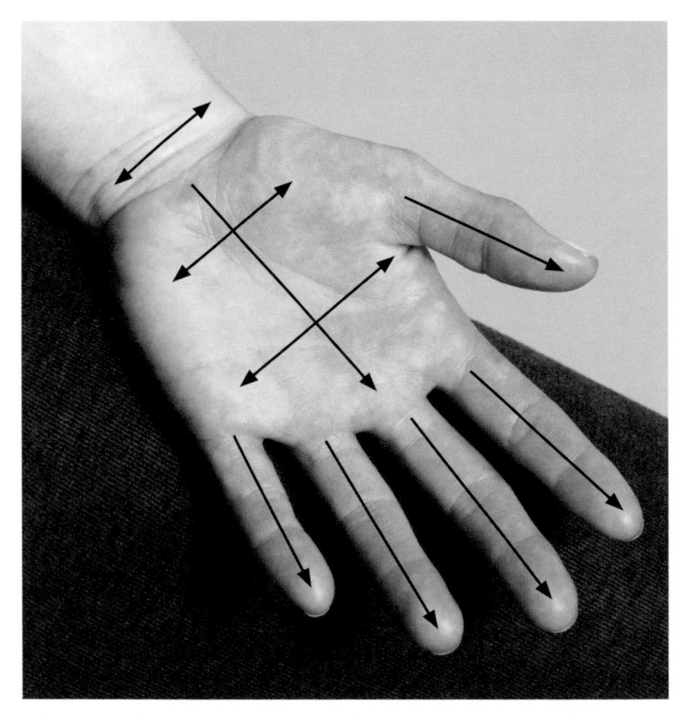

Allow your hand to open out to release contractions of flexor muscles. Think of your palm widening and fingers lengthening.

Exercise – Releasing thumbs

›› Our thumbs are very strong and are able to perform a myriad of complex movements. Consequently they can become very stiff and tense. Releasing tension in your thumbs can help your armpits, shoulders and the working of your entire back.

›› Sit down in a chair and position your bottom right back into the chair so you can lean against the chair-back or get vertical by sitting on your sitting bones. Free your neck and send your head upward. Place the back of your hand, palm upward on your upper leg. Allow your fingers and palm to release and open out as though they were spreading. Allow your thumb to spread away from your fingers, and let your fingers uncurl as they drop downward to your leg. Make no effort, but 'think' your hand to open out. 'Direct' the heel of your thumb within your hand to spread away from the palm. Think of your whole hand as softening or melting. As you release your hands, think of the space within your armpits opening up, let them breathe! Think wide across your shoulders and chest, but ensure you do not make effort nor 'pull your shoulders back'! Think rather than 'do'. This exercise can be performed anywhere, for example, on the bus or train, in a café or at home.

›› You can also encourage a release and opening out of your hands and thumbs by adopting a crawling position for a minute or more (see page 142).

Headaches and back pain

There are a great many causes of headache from dehydration to hormonal changes and stress and we should eliminate as many as we can. It is common for tension headaches to be caused by muscles tightening in our neck, pulling our head off balance and becoming fixed. This pattern interferes with our posture and is linked closely with back pain.

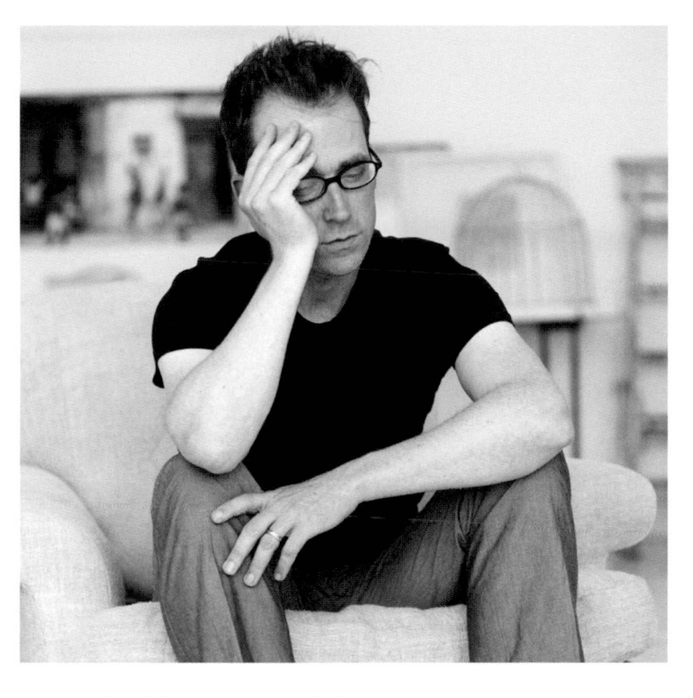

Exercise – Free your neck to avoid tension headaches

›› Neck tension is a common cause of headaches and we can do a lot for ourselves. Refer to the section 'Neck to be free' (page 74). Try to allow your head to roll forward a few millimetres on the very top of your spine, so you are not pulling it backward. Think of your head teetering. Allow your neck to release.

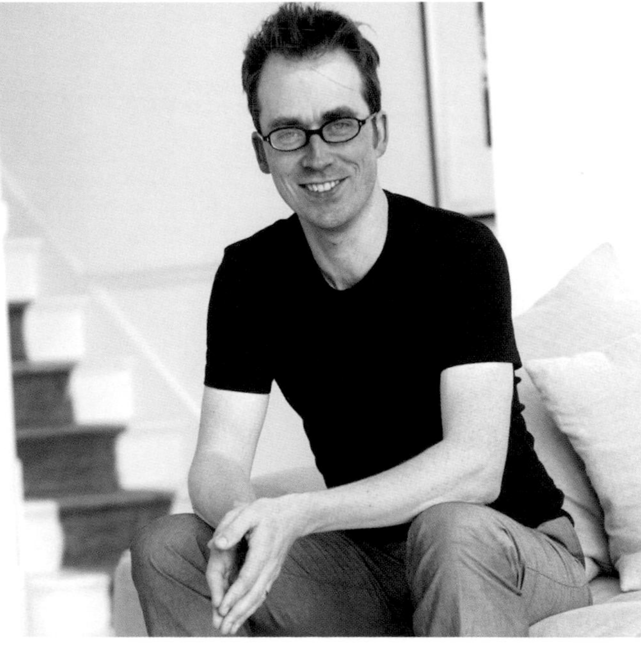

By releasing unnecessary tension in our neck and facial muscles we gain more freedom of movement and sense of reduced compression around our head. These releases can also benefit our breathing, blood circulation and the supply of oxygen to our brain.

t. *Headaches can cause us to pull down and shorten in stature.*

b. *Releasing your neck and shoulders can help avoid headaches.*

Releasing your lower back

There are a great many variations of habit that can affect our back, such as rounding our upper back (kyphosis), over-arching our back (lordosis) and twisting (scoliosis). It is impossible to cover all the variations of poor poise in this book, however the Alexander Technique principles will enable the appropriate natural curves of your spine to be restored by encouraging a lengthening and widening of your stature – all conditions required to avoid back pain.

HELPFUL TIPS

Here are some specifics you might wish to remember:

›› When standing, avoid pushing your hips forward so you arch your back. Turn side-on to a mirror to see if this is a habit.

›› Whether sitting, standing or walking, think of your head going forward and upward, your back lengthening and widening. Thinking of 'widening' your lower back helps make it stronger. Send your knees forward and away.

›› When sitting, allow the weight of your body to go down into the chair. Let the chair support you. It is very easy for us to 'perch' on the chair as though we were ready to get up at any moment. Think of your weight going down through your sitting bones into the chair. Release the muscles around your hips and pelvis. At the same time, free your neck and 'direct' your head upward.

Releasing your upper back

Upper back pain is frequently caused by hunching and loss of upright poise which in turn can cause distortion of the upper spine (kyphosis), compression of the discs and vertebrae, or an over-straightening of the spine.

In all cases, the procedure should be to 'inhibit' the muscular tendencies that are causing the distortion. It involves releasing unnecessary tensions and a restoration of the correct muscular co-ordination throughout the body. This is achieved by attending to the Primary Control (page 86), and giving directions to bring about healthy co-ordination. These should be applied first before any further considerations.

HELPFUL TIPS

›› If you have an over-straightened spine, you should endeavour to soften and release the muscles around the upper back and lie down frequently in Semi-supine Position. Give a great deal of thought to widening.

›› If you have an excessively curved and compressed upper back, much of your problem is probably linked to a tendency to shorten in front. We frequently talk of lengthening in our back but it is just as important to be lengthening in front. First free your neck, think of your head going upward then think of lengthening up in front so the distance from the groin to the Adam's Apple is lengthened, but avoid 'doing' anything such as arching your back in the process. Remember to 'think' and not 'do'. A release of tensions in the front of our trunk will enable us to lengthen and allow our upper back to restore its natural curvature.

›› Lying down frequently in Semi-supine Position will be of enormous help in releasing unwanted tensions in the upper back and this is discussed further in the following section.

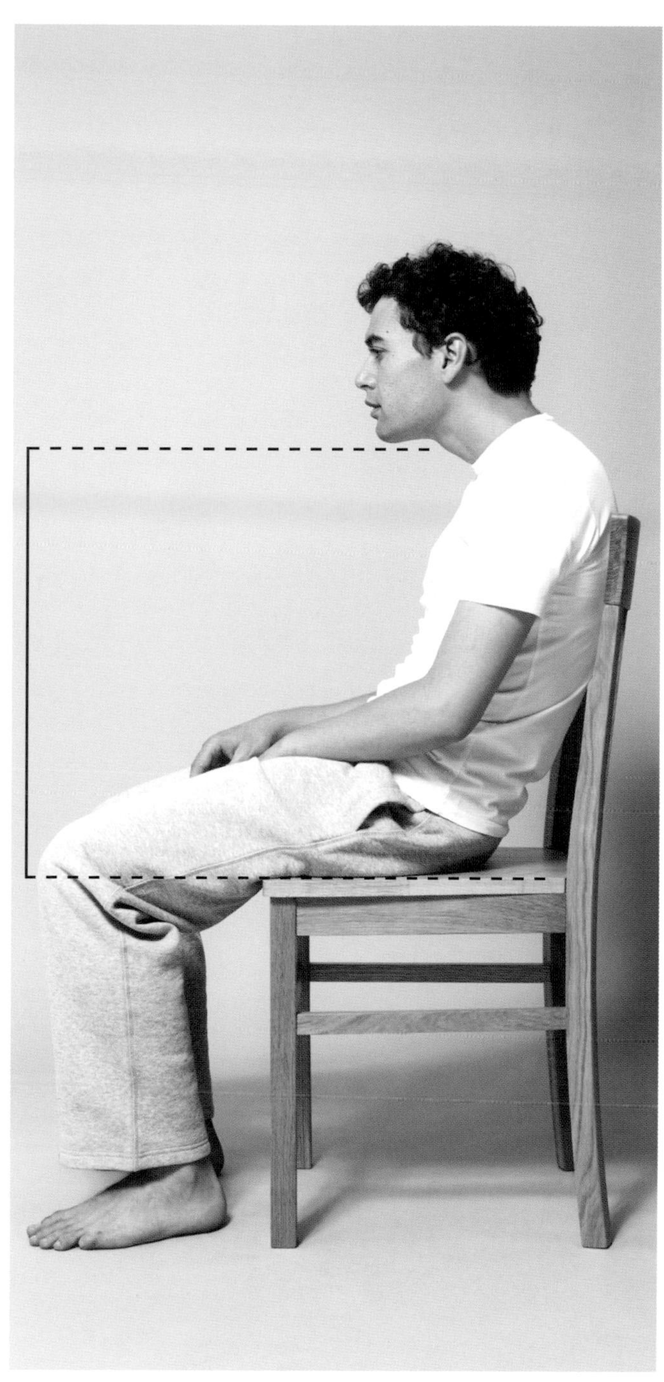

Slouching and stooping shortens our height and compresses our internal organs.

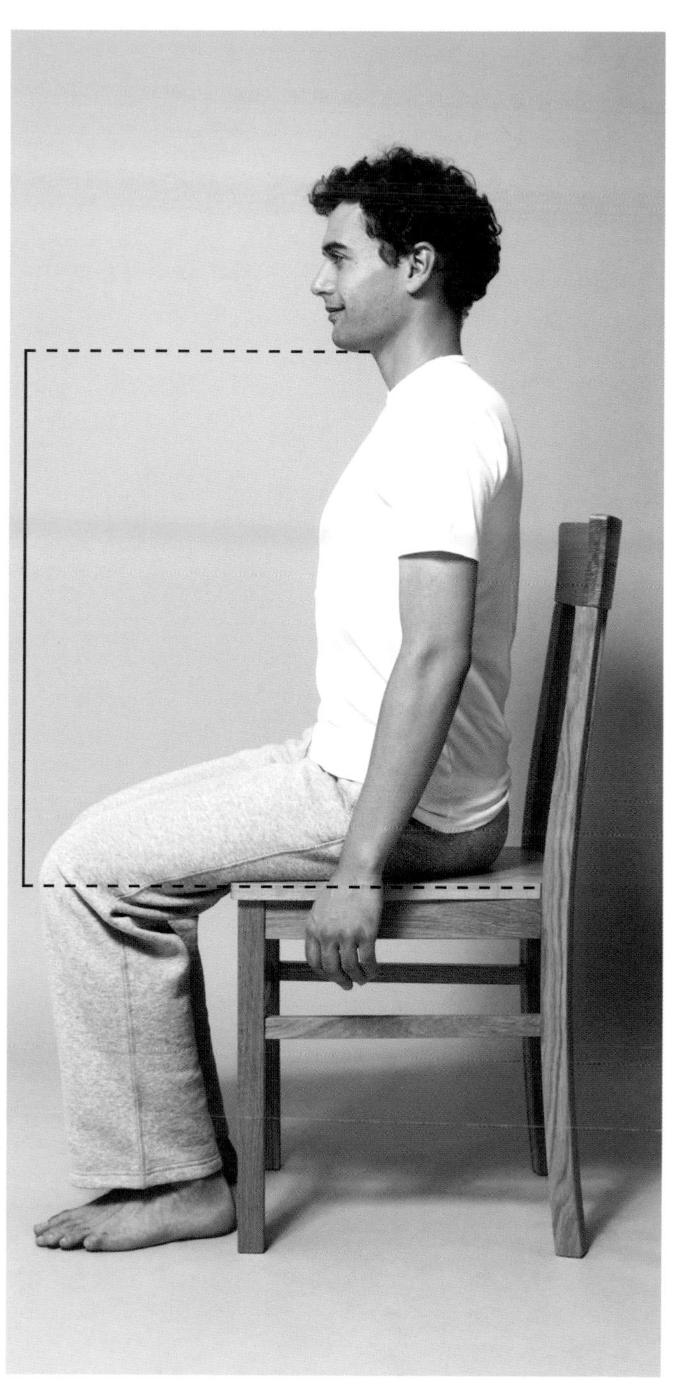

Lengthening helps to maximise our internal capacity.

Semi-supine Position

Lying down in Semi-supine Position is one of the most effective ways of restoring poise and ridding ourselves of unnecessary tensions. It is particularly helpful for people with back pain. When sitting or standing, our muscles are actively supporting us, but by lying down in Semi-supine Position we take the pressure off our spine and are able to release far more tensions by allowing gravity to have its beneficial effects on our back, neck, shoulders and pelvis. Our spinal and abdominal muscles are encouraged to release so our whole torso can lengthen and widen; our pelvis may rotate allowing our lower back to release tension and become flatter toward the floor; our diaphragm and the muscles around our ribs may release helping our breathing and reducing strain on our back. Our upper back is encouraged to straighten out, decreasing excessive curvature and increasing our height. This procedure is sometimes called 'active rest', as not only does it relax us but throughout the process we will be actively thinking to bring about positive changes to our co-ordination.

By lying down in 'Semi-supine' we give ourselves time to 'stop'. It allows our system to calm and become more still; it helps to reduce adrenalin and stress so we feel more refreshed. We can become more aware and conscious of 'holding on' to tensions so we can think of releasing.

Care should be taken to ensure we do not attempt to 'push' ourselves downward to flatten against the floor which would cause strain and stiffness. If you feel that your lower back or shoulders are not touching the floor, do not force them down. Allow gravity to do the job for you. If you can think of releasing or allowing yourself to melt downward, your body will gradually respond in a natural way.

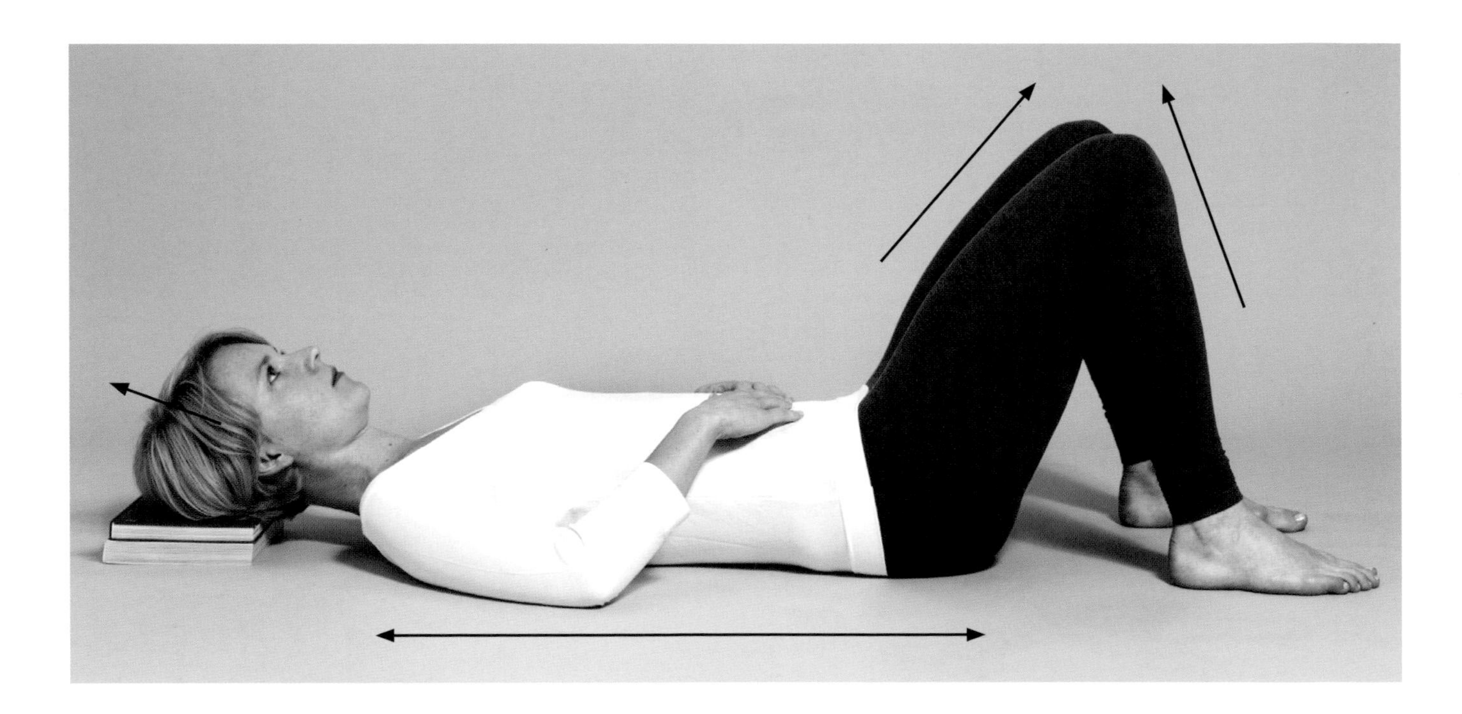

Exercise – Lying down in Semi-supine Position

›› Lying down in Semi-supine Position involves lying flat on your back on a carpeted floor, with your knees bent and a 5–8cm (2–3in) stack of books under your head (but not touching your neck). Your feet should be drawn up so your heels are about 45cm (18 inches) from your buttocks and spaced out about the width of your shoulders. Your elbows should be spread a little away from your waist and your hands should rest gently on your tummy. The books raise your head, tilting it slightly forward in relation to your spine, encouraging the release of tensions in your neck. You should lie in this position for around 10–15 minutes, and without doing anything physical think of releasing all tensions in your neck, shoulders, arms and lower back. As you think, you are communicating to all your muscles via the nervous system and this can have a profound effect on your well-being and posture.

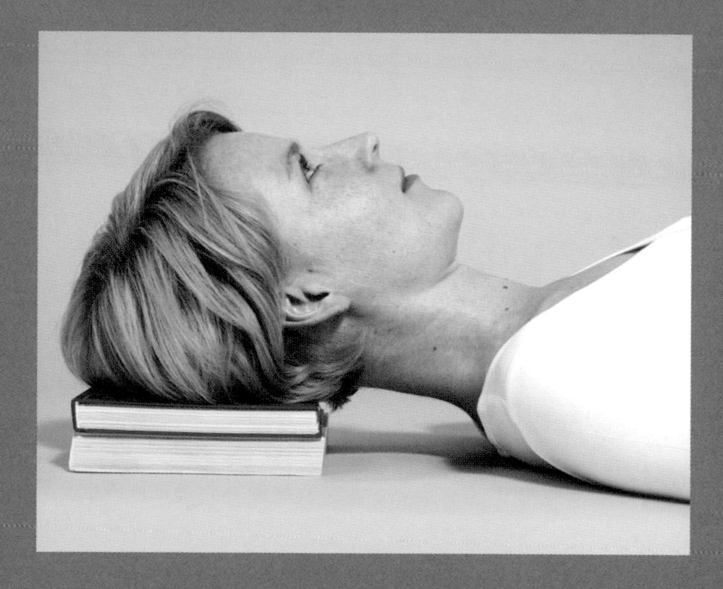

›› Endeavour to stay in the present and stop your mind from wandering. If you discover you have been thinking of something else, gently bring your attention back to yourself, lying on the floor and go through the following thought process.

›› The process of lying in Semi-supine Position can be performed in several phases.

1. Having lain down carefully in the manner shown so that your body is straight in alignment, just lie there still and bring your attention to your situation. Sense the nine points of contact you have with the floor: your head on the books, your two shoulders, both sides of your pelvis, your feet and your elbows all lying on the floor. Feel the weight of your body 'sinking' down into the floor.
2. Notice any unnecessary tensions that exist and think of releasing them. Allow your shoulders and lower back to 'melt into the floor'. Allow your hips to be free so your knees are simply balancing in an upright position pointing to the ceiling. Do not use effort, but think of doing less with all your muscles and allow the floor to support you. Ask for more release than you are normally familiar with. Think of releasing more than usual.
3. After a few minutes of releasing unwanted tension and just being still, we can begin to give directions to lengthen and widen. This is a thinking process and does not involve effort. Indeed any effort whatsoever will be counter-productive. As you are releasing, think the following 'directions':

- Think your neck to be free.
- Continue thinking 'Neck to be free' as you 'direct' your head away from your shoulders toward the wall behind you.
- Continue directing your head away from your shoulders as you ask your spine to lengthen.
- Continue directing your head away and back to lengthen as you ask your shoulders, middle back and lower back to widen and spread out across the floor.
- Continue with the above as you 'direct' your knees upward toward the ceiling. This gives them a 'purpose' and will enable them to balance freely in this upright poise without you holding on in your hips or ankles. 'Direct' your knees upward away from your hips and away from your ankles.

In all cases think the directions and make no effort. Think your directions, one after the other and all together.

Getting up from Semi-supine Position

1

When you get up off the floor, do not 'end-gain' by jumping up. Apply the 'means-whereby' approach so you retain the benefits of lying down. Follow this procedure for getting up off the floor:

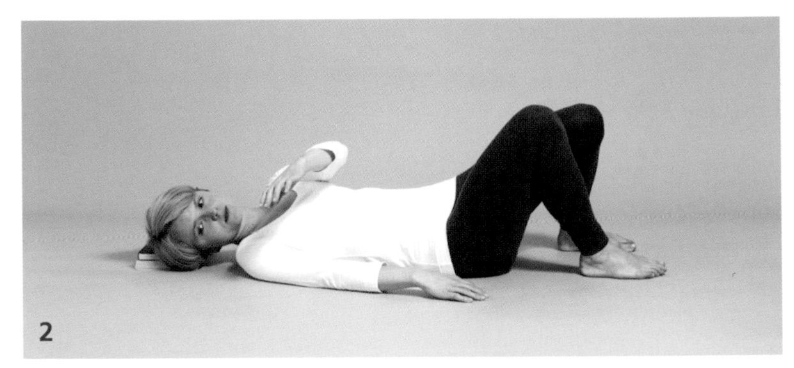

2

- Look to one side with your eyes and, as you roll over on your side, bring the opposite arm across you, leading with your fingertips, and place your hand on the floor. Keep your neck free all the time. (1–3)
- Bring yourself into a crawling position on hands and knees. Allow your back to be straight with face pointing toward the floor below you. (4)
- Sit backward onto your heels.
- Take your hands off the floor and bring your body upright while still sitting on your heels. Free your neck as you do. (5)

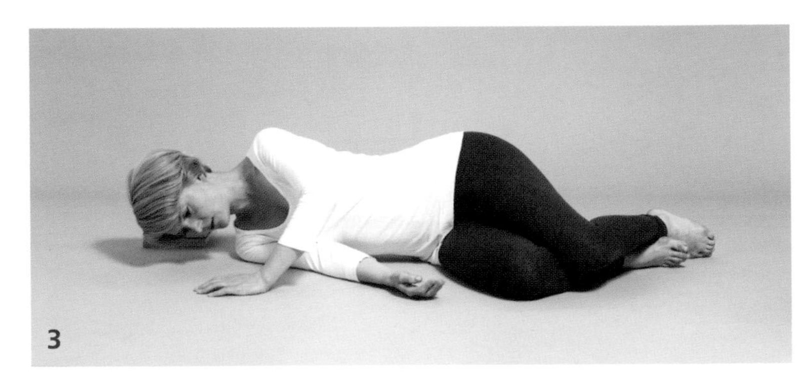

3

- Come up so you are now kneeling tall. Your body position will be similar to standing. (6)
- Bring one knee up so your foot goes flat on the floor in front of you. (7)
- Send your head upward over your foot so you end up standing. Put a hand on the back of a chair to steady you if you feel unstable.
- When you arrive in standing position, stop and centre your body weight over your ankles. (8)
- Free your neck by allowing your head to roll forward slightly. 'Direct' your head upward as you begin to walk.

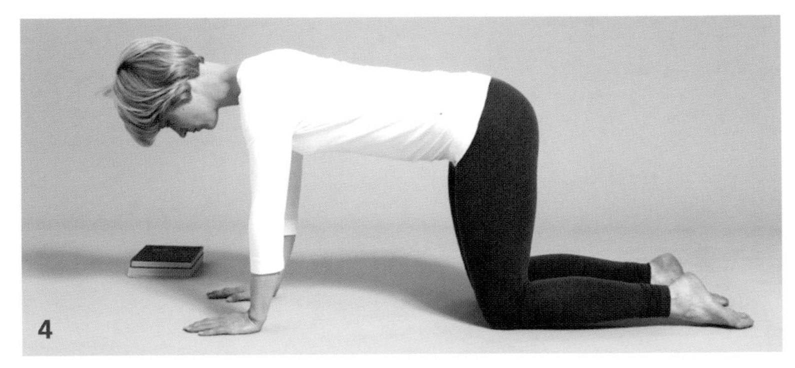

4

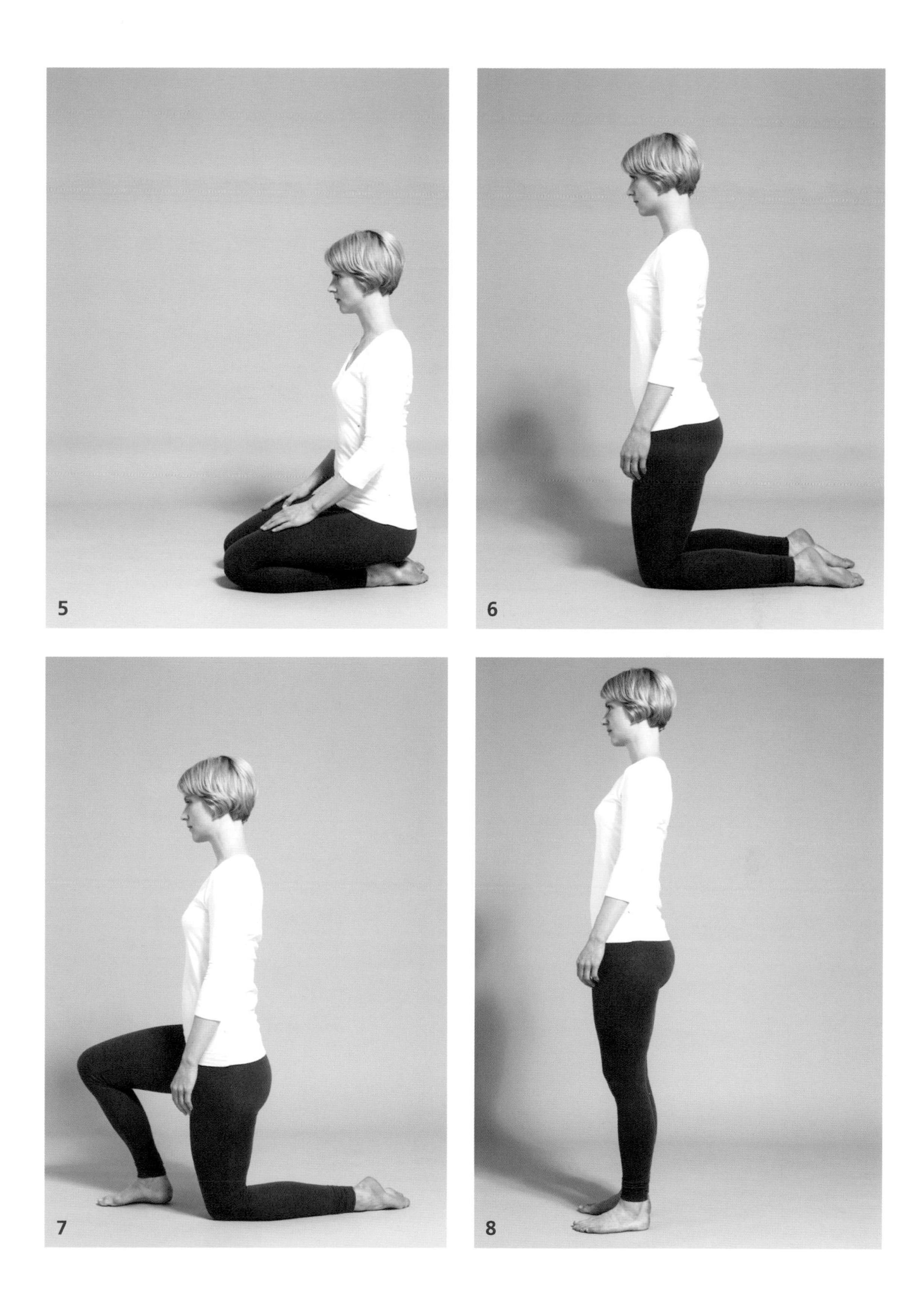
5
6
7
8

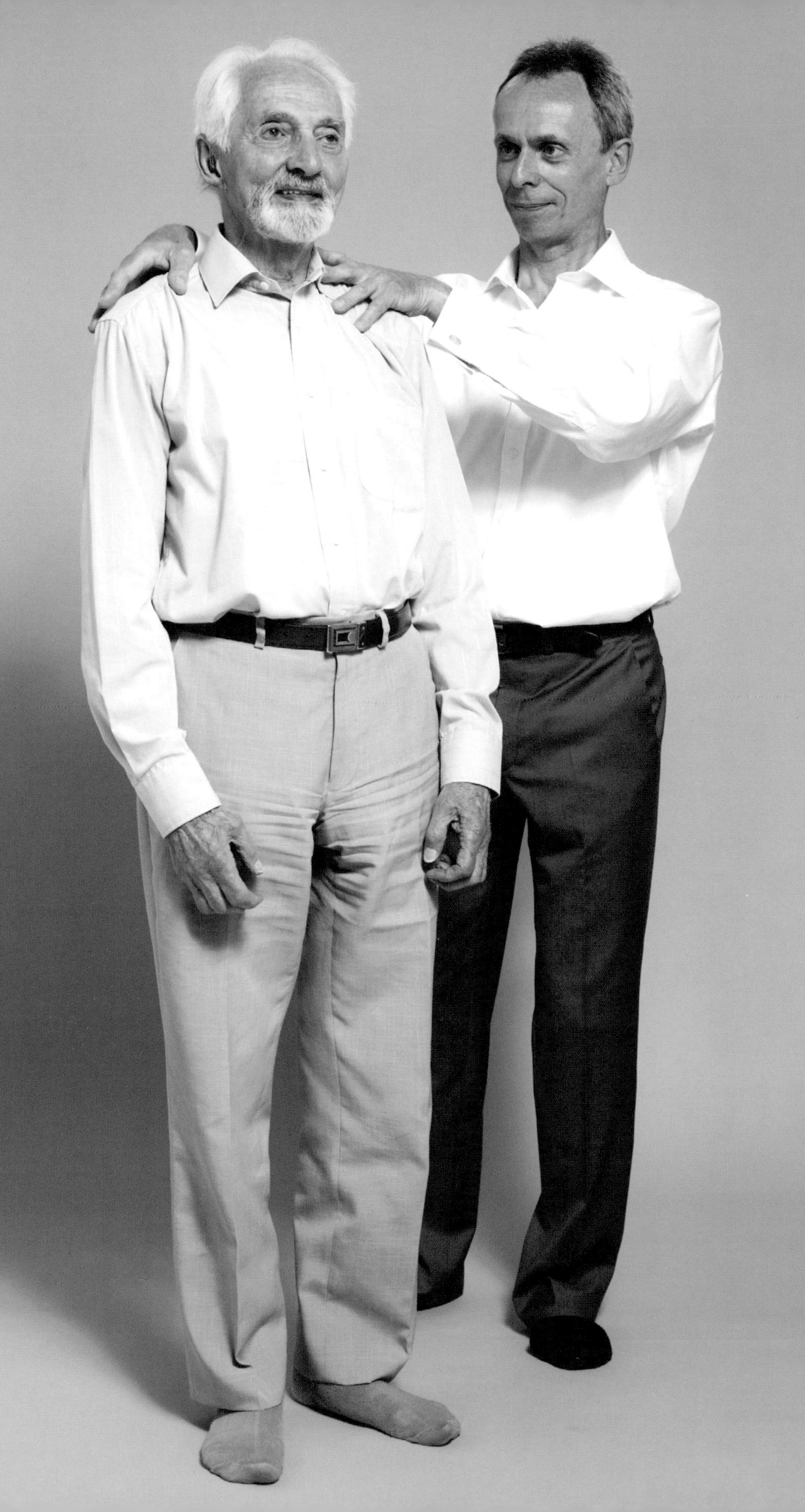

Learning later in life

The question is often asked, 'Is it too late for me to benefit from the Alexander Technique now that I'm over sixty?' The short answer to that is that it's never too late. Having worked with a great many people in their seventies, eighties and even some over a hundred years old, I can assure you that real changes and improvements to poise, balance and co-ordination can be made right into old age.

There are two main things working for us that enable us to change what seems like a lifetime of habits. First, no matter how ingrained our habits are from years of poor posture, they are not an intrinsic part of us. We have an instinct for healthy poise that we were born with and it remains with us throughout our life. Deep down, our body 'knows' what to do. We just need to allow it to work. When people say, 'you can't teach an old dog new tricks', my response is, you are never too old, and furthermore, you are not learning 'tricks'. If you were healthy as a child, the likelihood is that you had wonderful poise; you have experienced good posture before. This is re-learning the natural state that nature intended. The instinct is still there.

Second, you have very similar musculature to the time when you had healthy posture as a child except your size and proportions have changed. All the muscles and bones are still in the same place; you are still all living tissue and nothing has died off. What has changed is how you use your musculature during your daily life.

Your body is self-healing and by changing how you use your body, you will also change how it functions. By improving your balance and co-ordination you create the conditions under which your body can heal and better functioning can be restored, so we can enjoy being more active and fitter for longer. It is never too late.

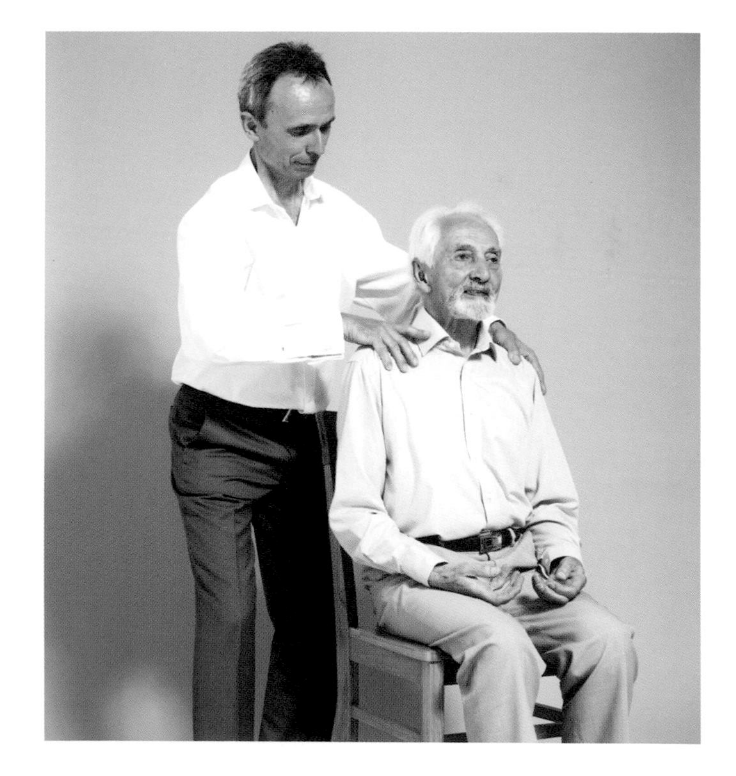

Having Alexander lessons later in life can improve our balance and agility while also reducing stiffness.

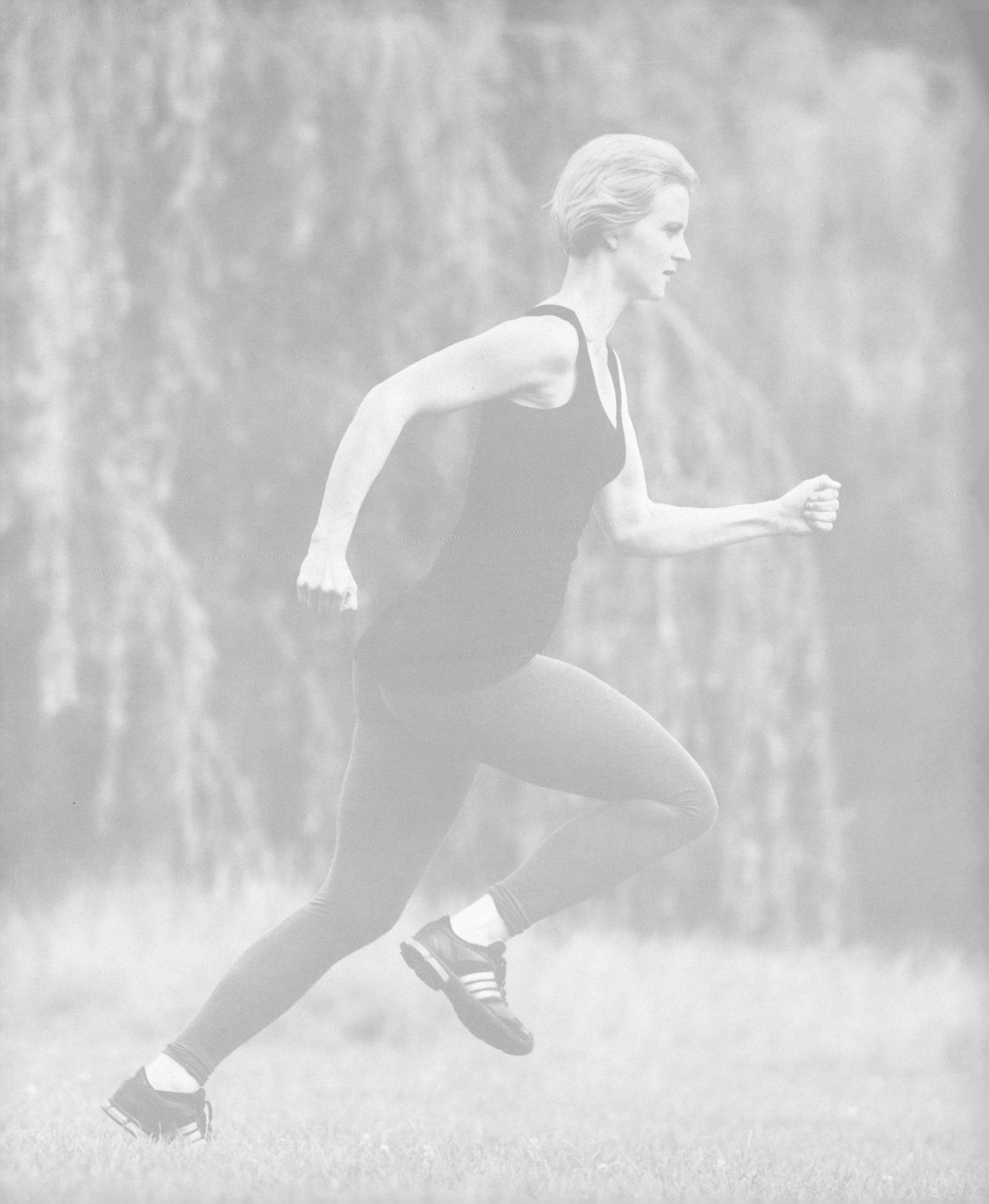

THINKING IN ACTION TO AVOID BACK PAIN

5

Release tension to move freely

It is usual to believe that movement only requires the use of certain parts of the body. So if we are going to walk, we use our legs or if we are going to bend we hinge at the main bending joints such as hips, knees and ankles. Well, this is all true, as far as it goes, but there is more to it than this.

Movement of any sort not only involves the use of certain mechanisms, but the body as a whole. Maintaining good Primary Control will help us move efficiently with correct direction. Preparing to make a movement usually causes us to activate many muscles in anticipation of the movement, but these tensions will be undoubtedly affected by our postural habits. We are most likely to over-use our muscles and cause unnecessary strain. So we should 'inhibit' our initial response to the stimulus to move and release. Ideally we should move from a point of stillness and avoid using any more effort than necessary. But even in stillness, muscles will be actively supporting us. I suggest that if we are going to begin an activity such as walking, we should first *cease doing the activity that precedes that movement*.

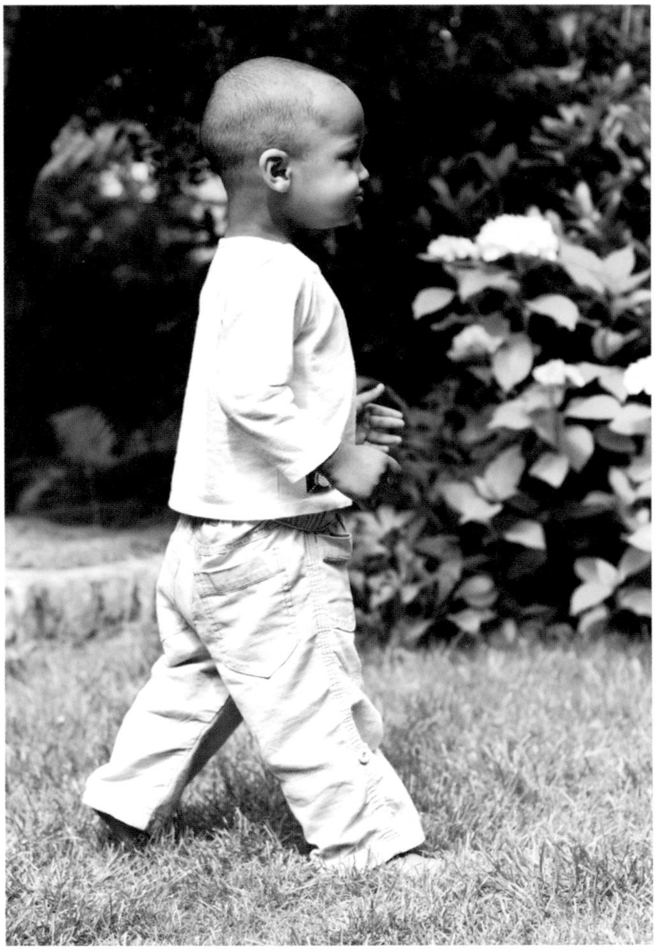

Child with free neck, lengthening in stature as he walks.

So if we are standing and decide to walk, we should release the muscles used for standing so that we can move forward easily. If we do not release our 'standing muscles' we will be fighting tension when we try to move. To bend, we should release the inside of all the bending joints – i.e. release in front of the hips, behind the knees and in front of the ankles – so they move freely, because when we are just standing, we are using muscles to support and stabilise these joints.

If we watch a toddler stepping forward, they will instinctively release their neck so their head nods forward a little, effectively putting it off balance but bringing about a natural lengthening of stature. They will then walk to catch up with their head! Now I'm not suggesting that we should be chasing around trying to catch up with our head all the time, but if we can release our neck first and allow our head to nod forward slightly off balance, we will initiate a lengthening of our back, which will activate our legs to walk or bend.

Giving directions during movements

The head leads and the body follows.

When we wish to move we do not want to lose the quality of light expansiveness that we achieve by giving our Directions. In fact we need this quality to help us move without any undue strain. So we should Inhibit moving instantly to give ourselves time to use a 'means-whereby' approach and think to prevent the wrong use. We can then release into the movement and continue giving Directions while we move. It's thinking in action.

Directions become the motive power behind our support system to enable us to move in accordance with our design. It is the way we have evolved. Our joints move more freely if the weight is taken off them just before the point of movement. We should release in order to move, and in order to do that, we need to direct our head upwards to bring about a quality of lengthening in our back as well as widening.

As discussed in Chapter 4, to move we should firstly free our neck, then 'direct' our head to go forward and upwards to lengthen and widen, activating our muscles in a well co-ordinated way so we are both supported and expansive. We then release the muscles around our bending joints so we move freely while maintaining the thought of 'going upwards'. We must 'go up' with our head to stand, we must 'go up' to bend, we must 'go up' to walk or to move anywhere. Going 'up' activates the support system.

Our body moves most efficiently if we are expanding as we move. It never works well if we shrink into ourselves, compressing our joints with tension and shortening our stature. Even bending downwards can be a 'lengthening' and 'widening' experience as it is the main bending joints of ankles, knees, hips that allow us to bend while also allowing us to keep our full height and width. Let us look at the Alexander Technique procedure of going into 'Monkey' which can help our ability to maintain an expansive, free quality.

'Monkey'

(a position of mechanical advantage)

Monkey Position, as it is commonly called, refers to a position that enables us to enhance how we 'use' ourselves. It is one of a number of 'positions of mechanical advantage', as F.M. Alexander called them. By moving into this position as a brief exercise, we can help improve our co-ordination, balance and poise by conscious control, which will benefit our 'use' afterwards. The process of 'going into Monkey' can both release joints and unnecessary tensions while engaging supportive muscles so we become expansive in stature, well supported and free to move, rather like a well-sprung angle-poise lamp. It is also a very efficient way of bending to avoid back strain. It can be used, for instance, when brushing your teeth, picking something up and while ironing.

The process of 'going into Monkey' may be practised once you have become familiar with Inhibition and Direction. It is a position that an Alexander Technique teacher will help you adopt, in order to bring about an enhancement of your poise, awareness, co-ordination and use of muscle. Indeed, it is a position the teacher may also adopt, to bring about the best 'use' of themselves while they are working on you!

Moving into 'Monkey' involves bending at all the main bending joints while also maintaining good balance and expansiveness throughout the body. It is a bent position that is neither standing nor sitting, but somewhere between the two, and can vary in height depending on your needs and wishes. The key considerations will be to move freely, in balance without shortening your stature. When you arrive in 'Monkey' you will remain free in your knees and hips and ankles so they are not gripping and the position is not fixed. As long as we are directing our head forward and upward and our back to lengthen and widen, support will be provided in an elastic and sprung manner that will enable us to be free and 'soft' in the joints so they are flexible and un-held and not compacted or tightened. Remember, the purpose of 'Monkey' is to work on our co-ordination. It is not a fixed position but a fluid poise that is infinitely variable.

In the following exercise I have broken the process of 'going into Monkey' into two stages. It is best to go through the procedure of Stage One several times over a number of occasions before attempting Stage Two. When you arrive in Monkey Position, only remain there a few seconds before returning to standing by 'leading the way with your head'. Practise the process of 'going into Monkey' several times as your ability and awareness will improve each time. Do not linger there longer than a few seconds. Once you are able to move into a Monkey Position that is balanced, free in your knees, hips and neck, you can add Stage Two to your exercise. You will then remain in the position longer, i.e. for 15–30 seconds or so, while giving directions.

Exercise – Monkey Position

Monkey Position is far more about preventing and inhibiting the wrong thing from happening rather than 'trying to do it perfectly'. If we avoid the interference of our habits, we will move freely and in balance. Pay particular attention to not stiffening your neck or knees.

Stage One

» Stand with your feet spaced slightly wider than your hips and turned slightly outward.

» While standing, observe your balance. Come back on your ankles a little and ensure you are not pushing your hips forward or leaning.

» Free your neck, 'direct' your head forward and upward, and your back to lengthen and widen.

» 'Inhibit' moving into 'Monkey'. Think of releasing in front of your ankles, behind your knees, in front of your hips, and release right up to behind your ears (the occipital joint).

» Before you bend, think it all again. Inhibit moving, release in front of your ankles, behind your knees, in front of your hips, and release right up to behind your ears, then allow your head to nod forward just a few millimetres to release your neck to initiate your movement into 'Monkey'. Think of your head going upward as you bend. 'Inhibit' pulling your head backward as you move.

» Allow your knees and hips to bend at the same time.

» 'Direct' your knees to go 'forward and away' over your big toes as you bend. Bend as far as halfway toward a chair, rather like skiing. The degree of bend in your hips should mirror the bend of your knees, so you are tipped forward from your hips.

» Avoid arching your back or sticking your bottom out. Also avoid collapsing your front; maintain the maximum distance from the groin to the throat as you bend. Ensure you do not drop your neck down; it should be aligned with your back.

» You are now in Monkey Position. Check that you are in balance, neither leaning forward nor backward.

» Release your knees so they are not gripping. They can be 'soft'. The quality of poise should be light and springy, (but do not bounce up and down!). Imagine sitting on a 'cushion of air'.

» Allow yourself to breathe.

» Come back up to standing again by leading the way with your head. Repeat a few times. Stop before you are tired.

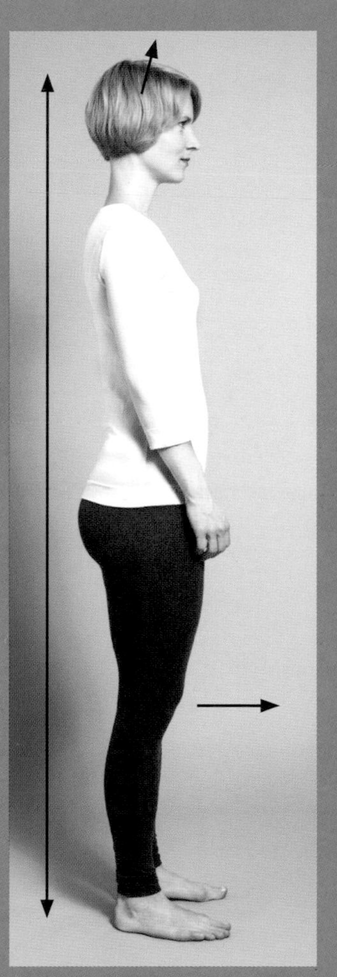

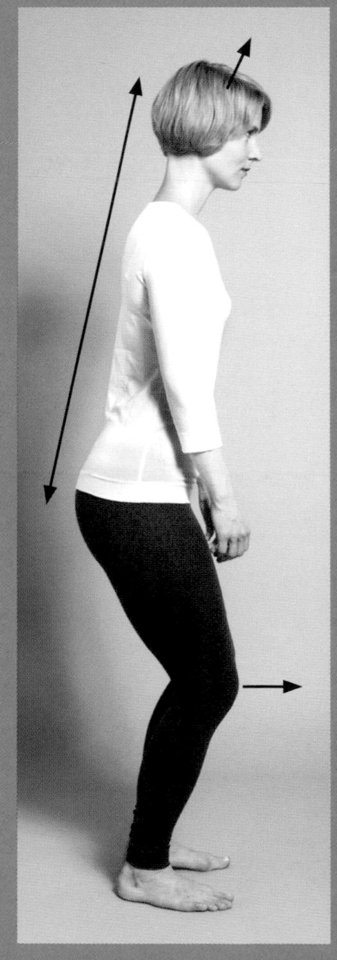

Stage Two

When you have practised 'going into Monkey' several times over a number of occasions so you can move fluidly without effort or strain, preferably with hands-on guidance from a teacher, you can add the following to further enhance your co-ordination and 'use'. You will now 'give your directions'. 'Inhibit' any tendency to 'push' or force the position.

Having moved freely into a well-balanced 'Monkey':

- Stop and free your neck again.
- 'Direct' your head forward and upward. The direction will be at an angle, possibly toward the top of the wall in front of you because you are tipped forward from your hips. 'Inhibit' any effort.
- Back to lengthen – think it.
- Back to widen – think wide across the front of your shoulders and chest too.
- 'Direct' your knees to go forward and away over your toes. Release them forward over your big toes but do not alter your height.
- Remain in this position for a few moments as you 'give your directions'.
- Go over all the directions again: Neck to be free, head to go forward and upward, back to lengthen and widen, knees to go forward and away.
- When you decide to come up standing, 'inhibit' first so you can choose to free your neck.
- Lead the way with your head as you come up to standing again.

Note: It is best to practise in frequent short sessions so you do not tire rather than undertaking one long session which can be counter-productive and even harmful.

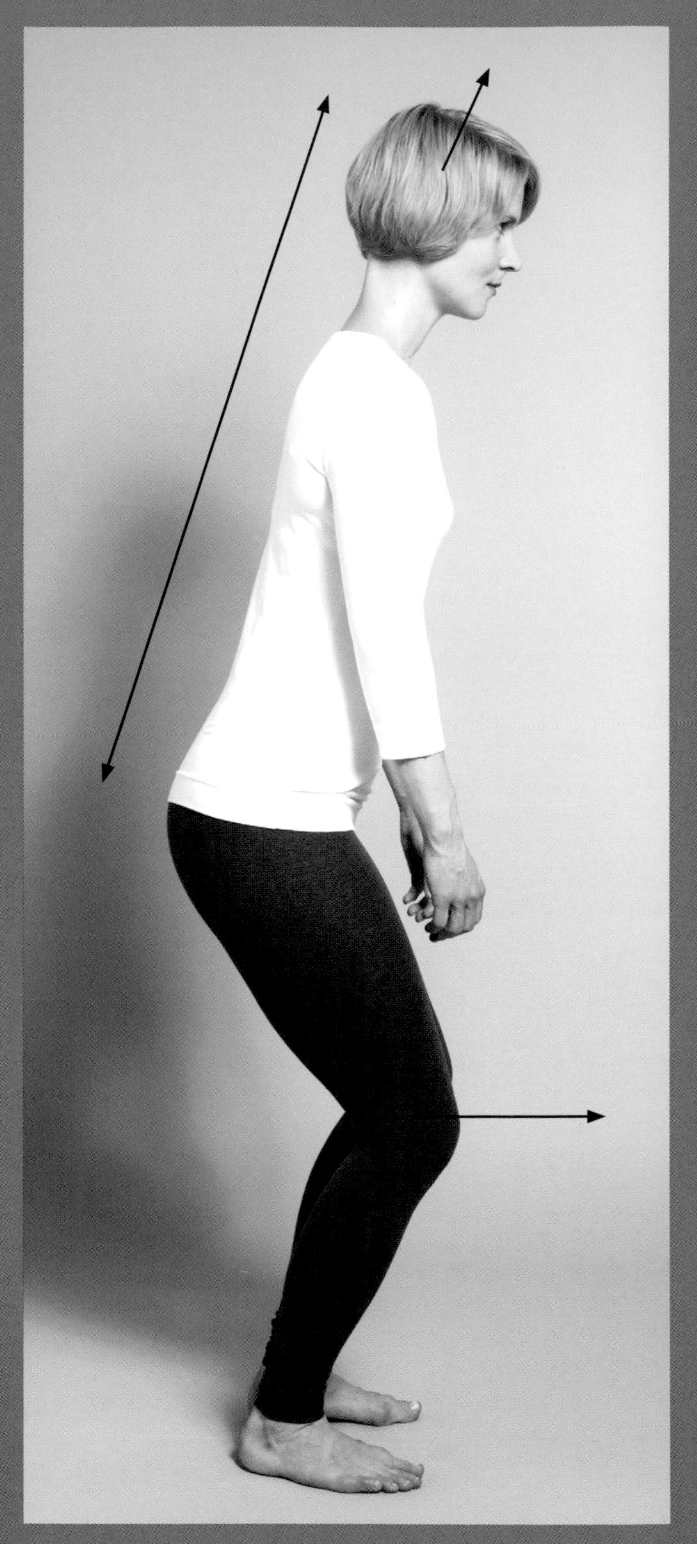

In Monkey Position your neck should be free, direct your head forward and up, and release your knees forward and away.

'Monkey' in action

Monkey Position is not only a procedure to help fine-tune our co-ordination but is also a most beneficial way of bending as it helps avoid unnecessary strain. Try to be free in movement, keep your neck free, let your knees bend forward over your big toes and never fix the position.

When your back is lengthening and widening it is well supported and you may be surprised how strong it can become. When your back is working well, your arms and legs will be able to make less effort when carrying and lifting, as they will be better connected and supported by your back muscles. Monkey Position can help train your back muscles to work in a well co-ordinated way when practised slowly and with care and observation.

HELPFUL TIPS

›› Free your neck first and think your head going upward when you bend and think your head upward when you return to standing.

›› Don't pull your head backward as you bend.

›› Don't let your neck loll forward. Your neck is a continuation of your back. Let your neck be free by allowing your head to roll on the top joint of your spine, not the lower joints. Think 'up' when you bend to help stabilise your neck.

›› Don't stick your bottom out. Release your knees forward and away.

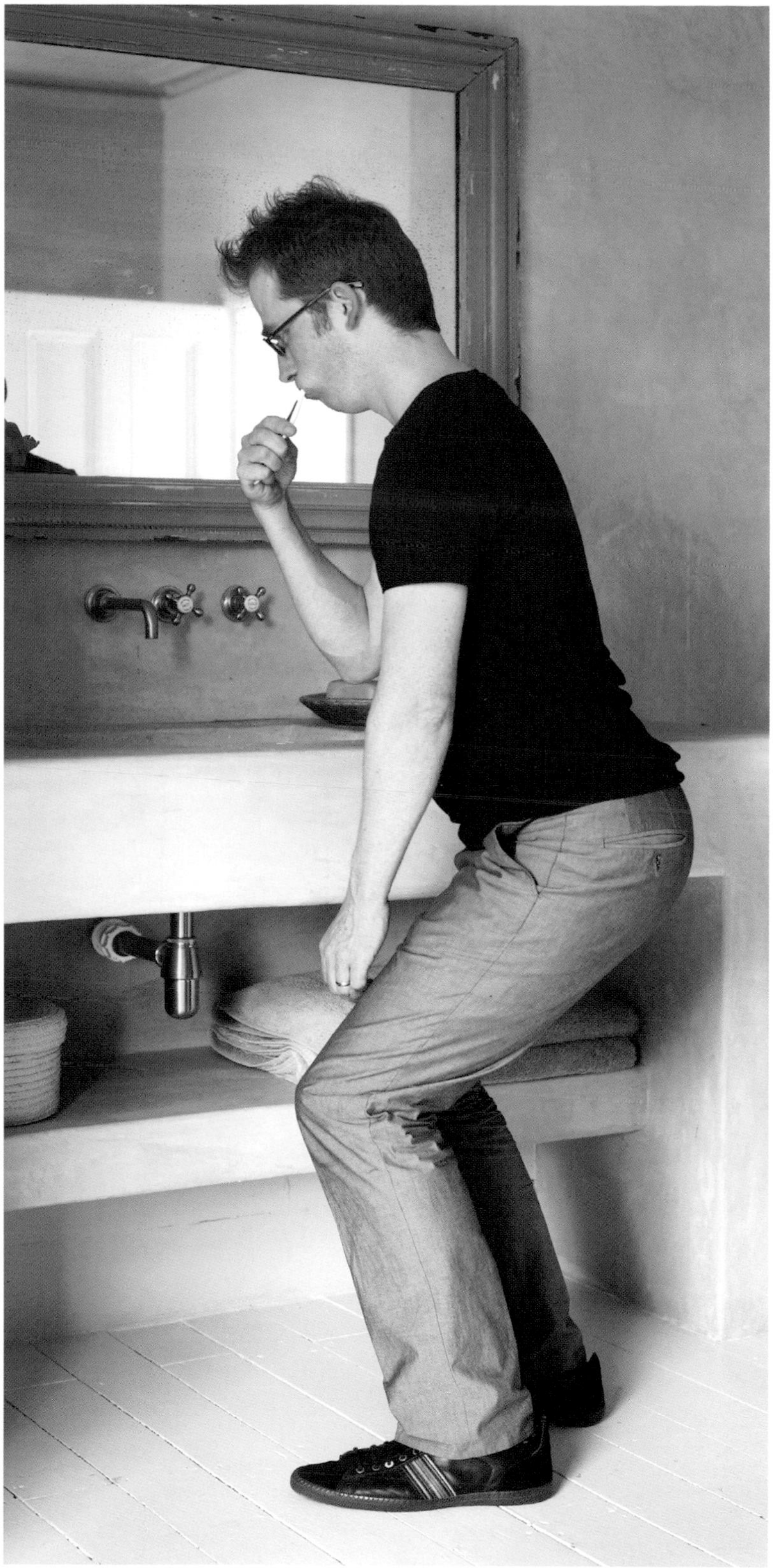

A good 'Monkey' is free in all the joints and in balance.

Standing without strain

One wouldn't think standing could be so difficult given we've got legs intended for the purpose. We learnt how to stand at the delicate age of 14 months and will do so until we are too frail to continue in old age. Yet the 'act' of standing can be fraught with problems, particularly if we have postural habits that interfere with the subtle co-ordination of our muscles. It is therefore quite common for 'standing' to literally become a real pain.

Let us look at what 'standing' actually means. It's common to consider 'standing' as holding ourselves upright on two legs, requiring muscle work in our legs and back. Any resulting tiredness and pain in these areas support this view. However, I would suggest that the 'act of standing' is an activity that involves the efficient and co-ordinated use of hundreds of muscles throughout the entire body. Our difficulties occur when we over-stiffen some muscles to compensate for the under-use of other muscles, causing a combination of collapse and stiffness.

Within our body we have what we could call postural muscles; an arrangement of muscles throughout the body primarily using red fibres that will support us tirelessly. These red fibres are fed on oxygen and intended for prolonged use in providing postural support and, as they are nourished by oxygen, are refreshed with every breath we take. On the other hand, white fibres, which we need for short strenuous bursts of activity are fed on glucose and tire quickly. Postural habits interfere with the efficient use of the red fibres, causing us to compensate by over-using our white fibres, so consequently we feel tired quickly by standing.

Our body's musculature is 'designed' to provide support yet still allow for expansive stature and freedom in the joints for movement. The Alexander Technique addresses the co-ordination of all our muscles, so they work efficiently as intended, improving the use of our red-fibred postural muscles. Our whole musculature is brought into the necessary finely-tuned co-ordination by our 'need' to be at full height.

There are two influences that will bring about healthy upright poise.

1. Gravity and the pressure of the floor under our feet activate our postural reflexes. Our body responds to the pressure on the soles of our feet.
2. Our 'need' as an individual to be 'going' upward to our full height activates the postural muscles. This can be seen in young children as they are gregarious and expansive in personality and stature. Their wish is to be tall like Mummy and Daddy and this 'wish' to be tall activates their musculature. As they do not have postural habits their combination of red fibre and white fibre muscles are working in a well co-ordinated manner so the 'act of standing' is effortless.

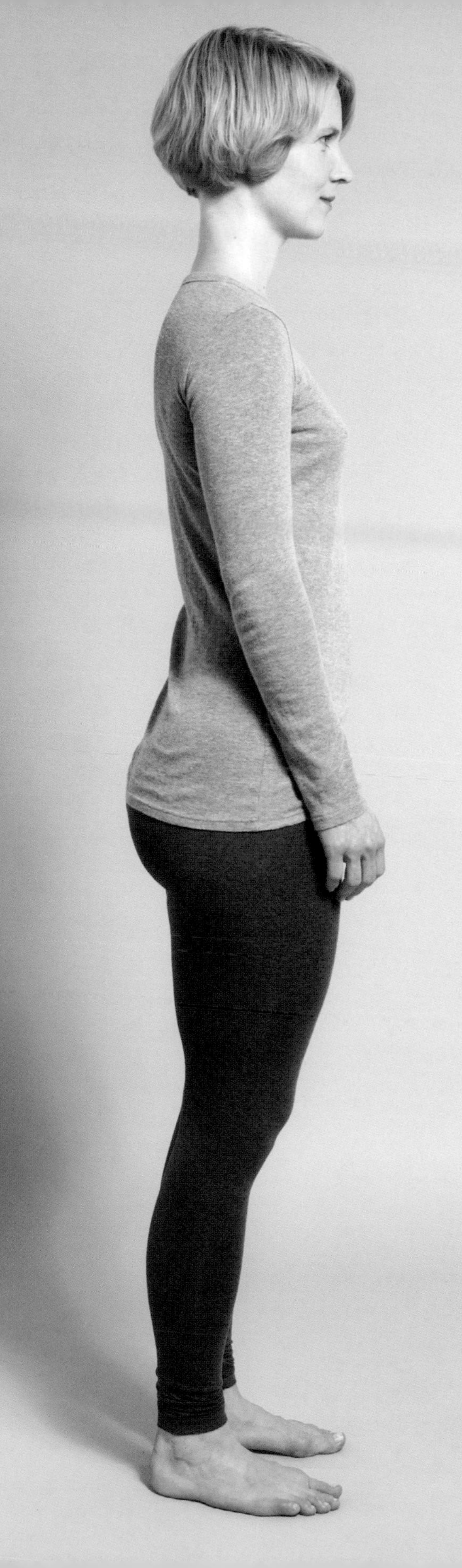

Pain-free poise occurs when all the muscles throughout our body are working together in good co-ordination. This requires our neck to be free, our head to be 'going' forward and upward and our back to lengthen and widen. Do not stand with your hips pushed forward or arching your back. Your legs should not be braced or stiffened and your knees and ankles should not be locked in position; your joints should be free. Indeed the quality of co-ordination you want is the same as for any other activity. When you are 'going up' the muscle tone exists to support you and in this respect, the 'act of standing' could be considered as not sitting or squatting!

There are three weight-bearing points of the foot: behind the big toe, behind the little toe and under the heel. Our body weight passes through our legs and ankles then spreads out across the arch of each foot to the triangle formed by these points. When standing we should have a sensation of being more over our heels than the front of the foot. However there should be no tendency to tighten the toes or lift them off the floor. Let your toes lie freely and allow the whole foot to 'soften'. Let your weight go down 'into' the floor so you feel grounded. This gives a firm base from which to think of lengthening upwards.

Free your ankles so there is a little sway available to help discover upright balance. Experiment with the exercise on page 48 called Faulty Sensory Perception.

In order to enjoy standing without strain we should never get fixed in position. To remain free and vary the weight distribution through your legs and feet to avoid tiredness, try the following exercise.

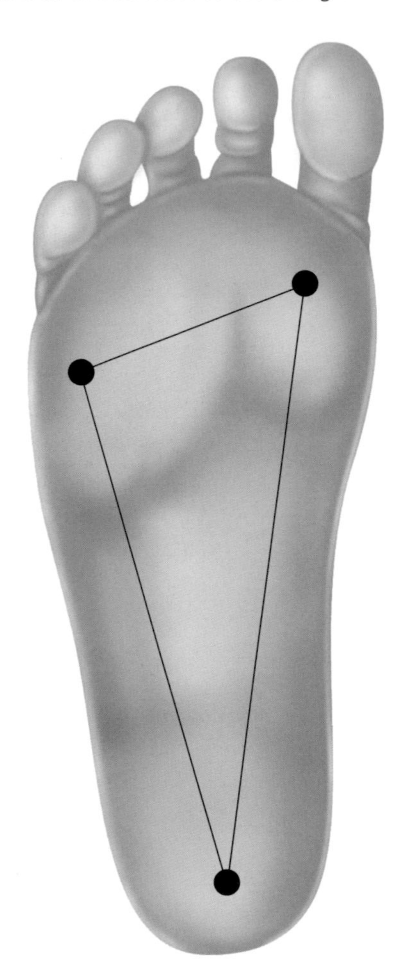

There are three weight-bearing points in each foot, and the arch between them acts as a spring.

Exercise – Standing with one foot advanced (mini-lunge)

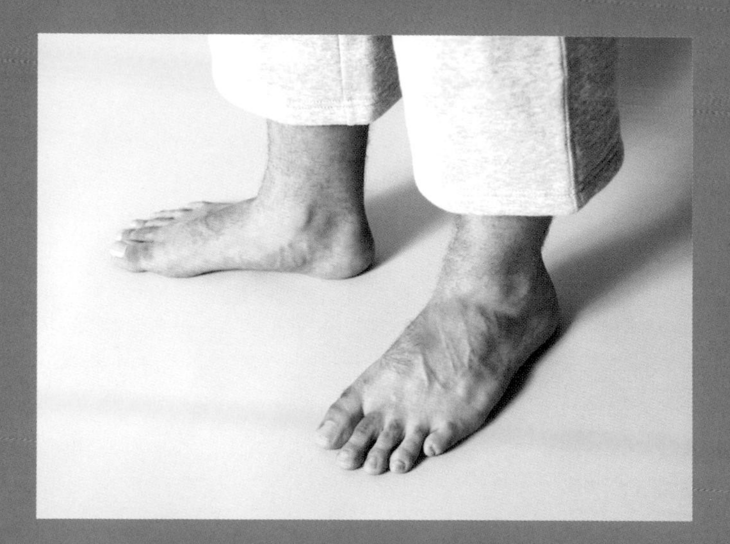

- Stand with both feet spaced so they are under your hips and turned slightly outward. Free your neck by letting your head nod forward a few millimetres, 'direct' your head to go upward and your back to lengthen and widen. Bring your weight back so it is more over your ankles.
- In a moment you are going to move one foot very slightly forward so that it is half the length of your foot in front of the other and turned slightly outward. But first, 'inhibit'. Stop to think of freeing your neck first and 'direct' your head to go upward to lengthen in your back. Then take a very small step of only 10cm (4in) forward and sideways. Lead the movement with your right knee at the same time as your head is going upward.
- Now you have one foot slightly advanced in front and to the side of the other like a mini-lunge position (see Lunge page 140)
- In a moment you will slowly transfer the weight of your body from the heel of the rear foot to the heel of the foot that is advanced, so your body weight moves very slightly forward and to one side. But first 'inhibit', to think of your neck free and head 'going' upward over your other foot. 'The head leads and the body follows.'
- Having moved your body weight forward, you can now move back over the other heel by first 'inhibiting', then freeing your neck, 'direct' your head upward as you move back. The degree of movement will be very slight and barely noticeable by anyone else.
- Sway backward and forward very slightly to experience how you can vary the weight distribution of your body to avoid becoming fixed in a position. You can do it in a bar or the post office queue!
- Try the same exercise by moving the other foot. Follow the guidelines above. 'Inhibit' first to think before you move.

Sitting without strain

Sitting is one activity we are required to do for hours at a time, yet prolonged periods in a chair can often cause backache, neck tension and even lethargy and stress. Let's face it, our body is much better designed for movement, but if we are going to sit we should endeavour to do so in the best way to avoid unnecessary strain.

Although we may have an adjustable office chair at work, during our lifetime we will sit on thousands of different styles of chairs, so it will be helpful if we can look after ourselves, rather than rely on chair design, to help avoid back pain. It only requires us to be aware and to think of how we sit.

It may be surprising, but a chair with a firm seat and fairly upright back is better for sitting in than a soft and squashy sofa. Although, with a little care, we can be comfortable on very soft sofas too.

When sitting, try to ensure that you are on your two sitting bones which protrude from the underside of your pelvis. You can locate these by sitting on your hands, palm upward and reaching right underneath until you can feel two bony protuberances. These are your sitting bones which take the weight of the body as we sit. If we collapse our back and slump, our pelvis rotates underneath us so we end up sitting on our sacrum. So it's important to be lengthening upward, leading with our head in order for our lumbar curve to assume its natural curvature and then we will be more on our sitting bones. Our legs join our pelvis at the side where the head of the femur locates into the socket, so when we are sitting, we are not sitting on our legs although the leg muscle may be touching the chair. 'Direct' your knees to go forward and away when sitting to help to release unwanted tensions and de-compact your hip joints.

To encourage our back muscles to support us without strain, we need to ensure they are co-ordinating together properly. We achieve this by using the Alexander Technique directions when sitting or standing.

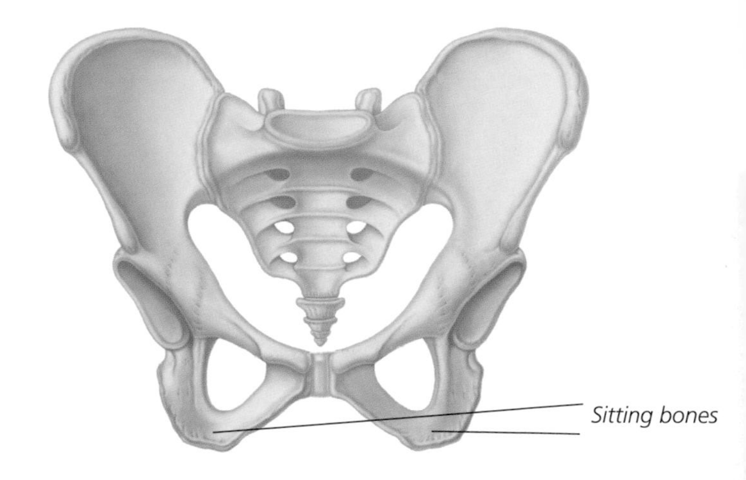

Pelvis – showing sitting bones.

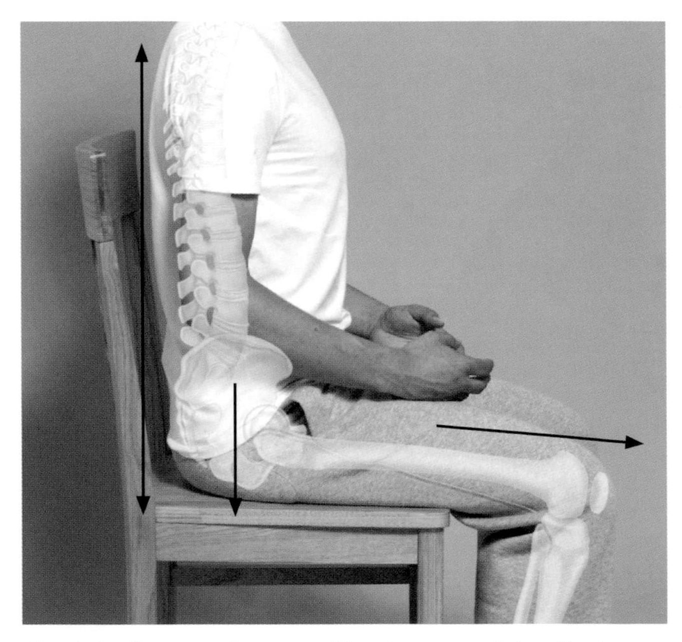

The sitting bones under your pelvis take your weight, allowing your legs to be free.

The key to sitting comfortably and avoiding problems is to always be in balance and allow your weight to pass through your sitting bones. By directing your head upward and your back to lengthen and widen, you encourage your muscles to support you without strain. Do not make a physical effort and avoid 'holding the position' as this will make you stiff.

Move frequently to avoid rigidity. When sitting we should ensure we never get fixed in a position. The quality we need is one of freedom, flexibility and expansiveness. You will be supported without any sense of effort if you are mindful to check you are not doing the wrong things and also if you 'direct' your head forward and upward; this thought engages the correct supportive muscles.

Note: You will not be able to sit upright all day and you should not endeavour to do so. Use the back of the chair regularly to give you support, and vary how you sit. Do this by bringing your bottom right back in the chair so you are as close to the chair-back as possible. A firm cushion is a great aid if positioned behind your lumbar and middle of your back. Your feet should be flat on the floor.

Exercise – Moving from standing to sitting

- To ensure good balance when sitting, we should endeavour to move into the chair in a free and balanced manner, with minimal of effort.
- Choose an upright chair with a firm horizontal seat so you can feel your sitting bones. The height should be roughly the height of your lower leg so when sitting, your thighs are parallel to the floor or slightly sloping downward.
- Stand in front of the chair with your feet spaced the width of your hips.
- 'Inhibit' sitting down to give yourself time to think.
- Do not consider 'sitting down' as a 'going down into the chair' exercise, but an opportunity to lengthen in stature as you bend at your hips and knees.
- Stand centrally so your weight is evenly distributed over both feet. Free your neck, think of your head going upward and your back lengthening and widening as you move.
- Let your knees bend so they go forward over your toes at the same time as you bend in your hips like a hinge. Keep your neck free and 'inhibit' the tendency to pull your head backward.
- When you arrive in the chair, 'inhibit' straightening. Pause a moment to sense your weight on your sitting bones. Allow yourself to come upright without rounding or arching your back. 'Direct' your head upward as you become vertical. Release your neck and shoulders. Let the weight of your head pass through your spine to your sitting bones in vertical alignment. Allow your feet to rest flat on the floor in front of you. Find your balance over your sitting bones. Let your hips be free so your legs are freely able to move from side to side.
- You can also sit further back in the chair in the same way, so that the chair-back or cushion supports you.
- When sitting it is important not to get stuck in one position. Sit freely and change your position by moving backward and forward from your hips (see page 119). Get up regularly to move around, fetch a glass of water.
- Avoid collapsing your lower back or allowing your pelvis to roll under you. Remain on your sitting bones, free your neck and send your head upward in your thoughts.

(See next page)

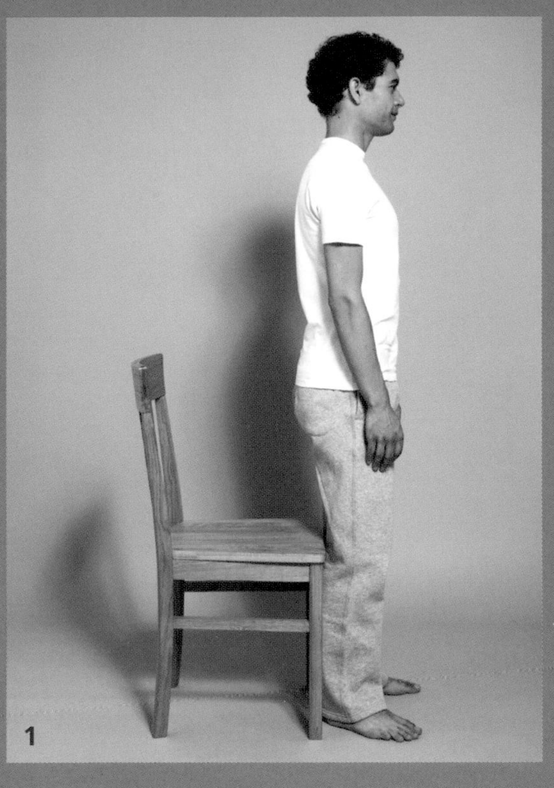

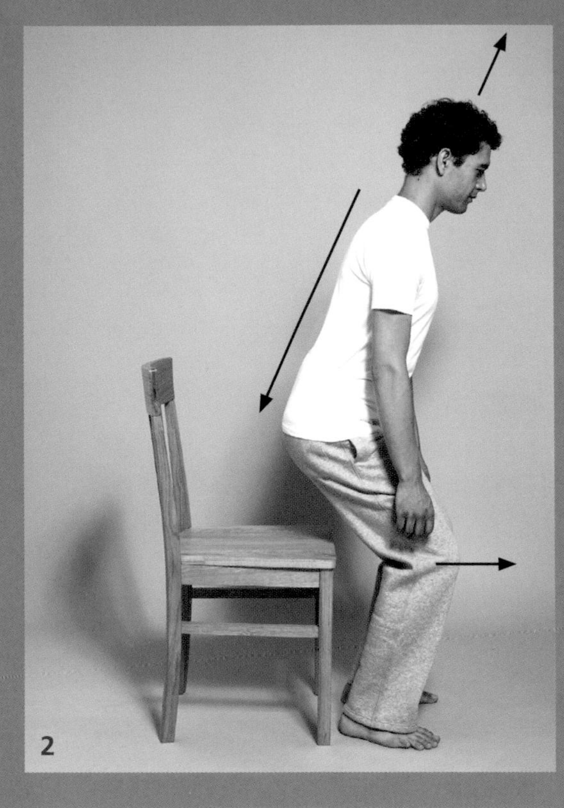

1. Firstly inhibit moving. Weight over ankles. Free your neck. Direct upwards.

2. Let your head roll forwards to start the movement. Let your knees go forward and away over your toes.

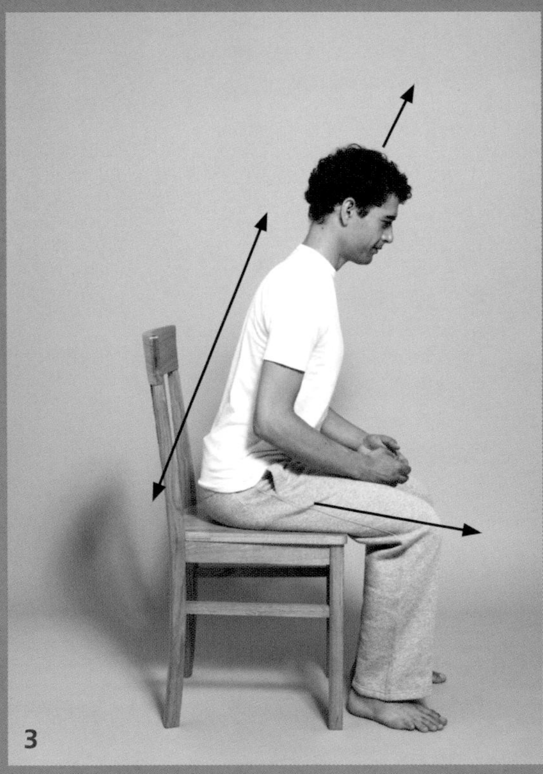

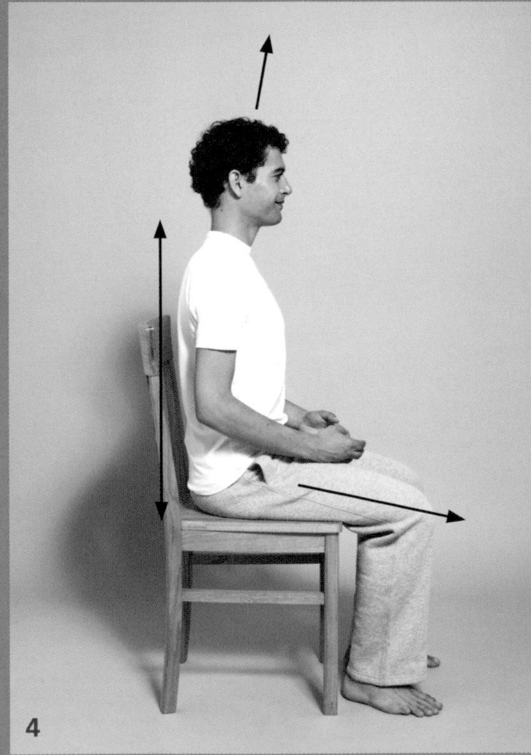

3. When you arrive in the chair, pause to direct upwards. Hinge back from your hips.

4. Feet flat on the floor. Give your directions to lengthen and widen.

Exercise – Leaning forward when sitting

A common movement we all need to do when sitting is to lean forward to reach something, either across a table or a desk. The movement also helps avoid getting stuck in one position.

- First, 'think' upward so you are upright and sitting on your sitting bones.
- Your feet should be flat on the floor in front of you.
- The important thing to remember is that you are going to lean forward from your hips, while maintaining a tall back. In other words, your back is not going to 'round' or collapse. If you are sitting in good balance, you will have a gentle lumbar curve and this will remain consistent as you move.
- Now 'inhibit' to give yourself time to think.
- Allow your head to fall very slightly forward on the top of your spine so that it is off balance. When this occurs you will be continuing to think of your head 'going' in a forward and upward direction so you lengthen in your back.
- Release in the front of your hip joints and the gluteus maximus (the muscle we sit on) to allow the movement. As your head rolls forward, slightly allow the weight of your head to take your whole body forward. Your head leads as you allow yourself to lean forward from your hips by 30cm (12 inches) or so with your body moving in 'one piece'. Hinge like the lid of a box and keep your back long. You must be free in your hips and truly sitting on your sitting bones so that you are able to move without stiffness.
- Before you return to upright, free your neck, think upward and come back in one piece.

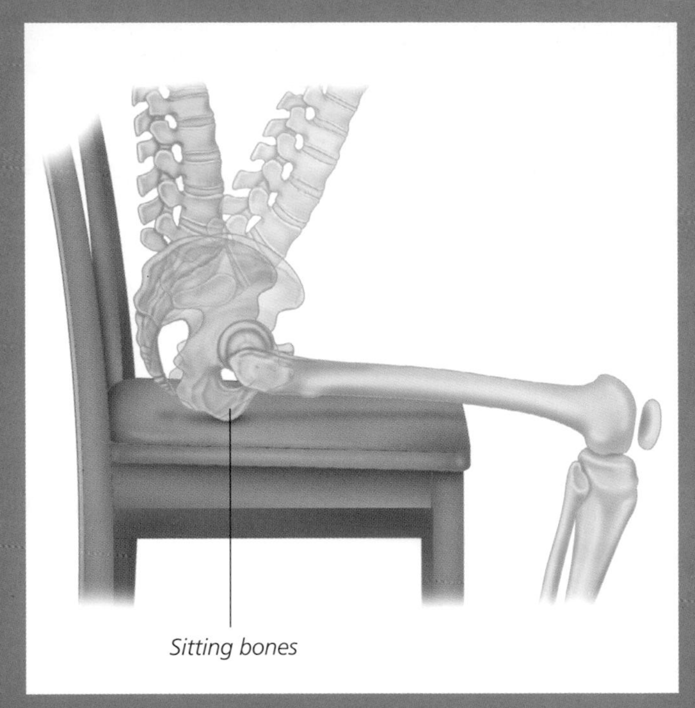

Our sitting bones take our weight. Pivot forwards from your hips to lean.

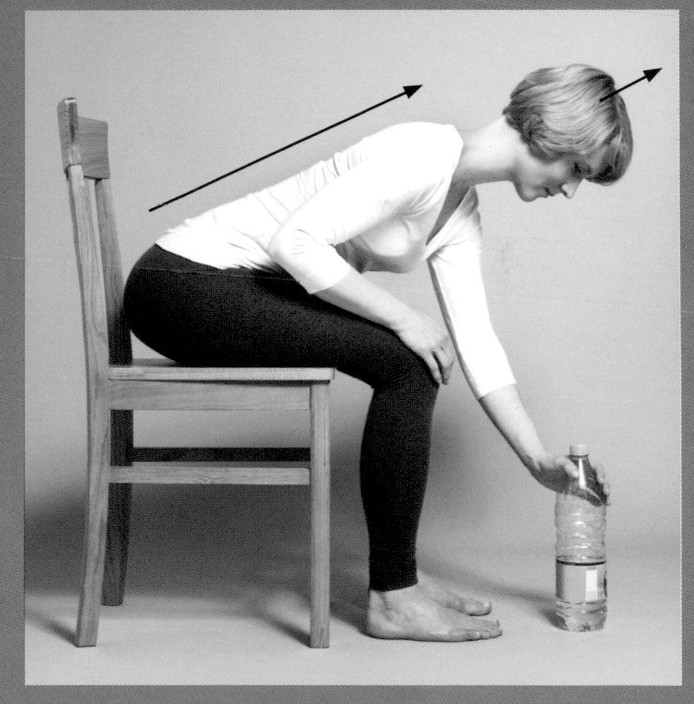

Hinge in your hips to bend and lead the way with your head.

Sitting reading

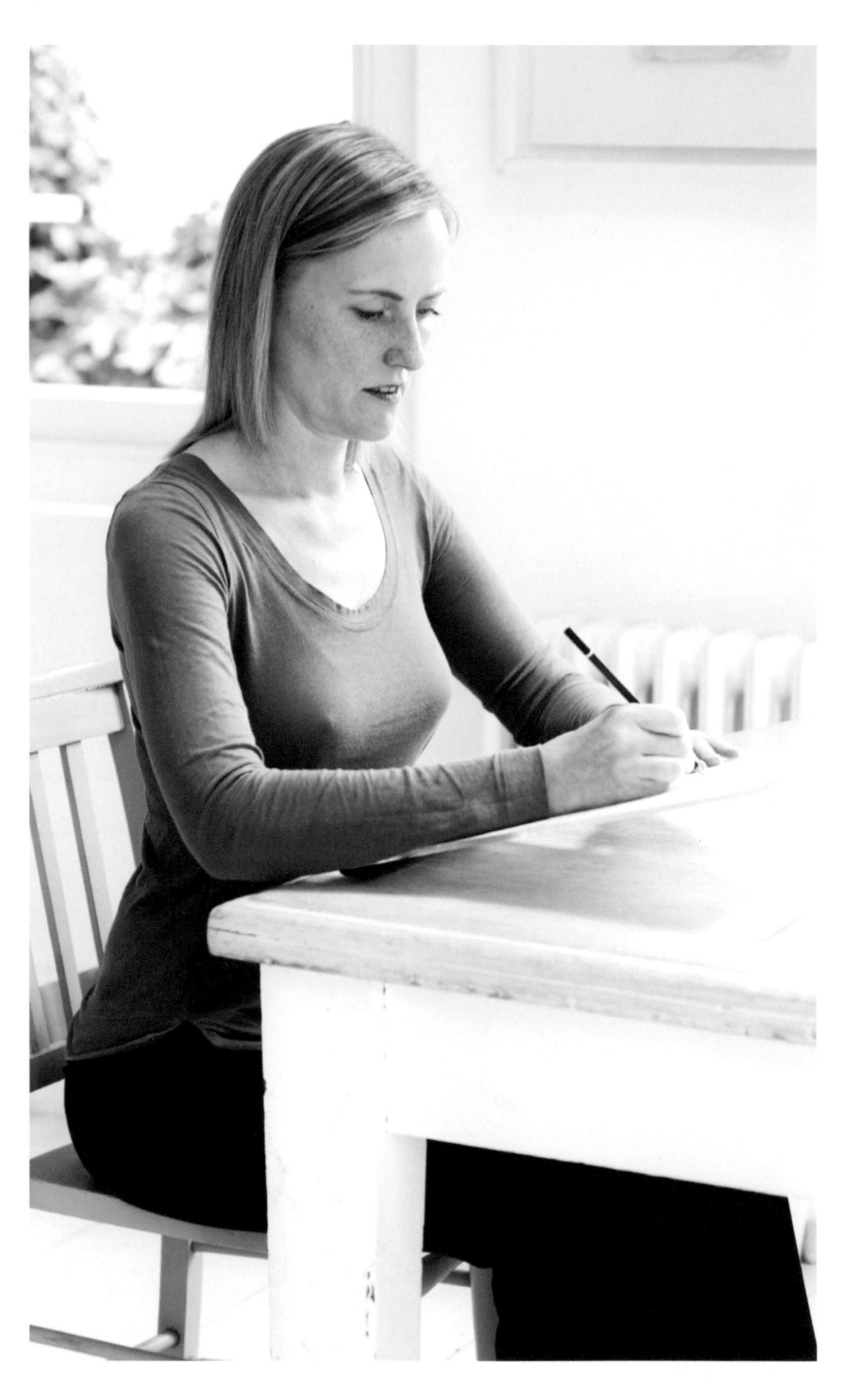

The problem with reading is that we tend to get drawn downward toward the book, paper or screen; it acts as a magnet and without awareness we have soon slouched or stooped, rounding our back and come off balance so we are under strain.

In order to read comfortably without causing back pain, we need to raise the book up to reduce distortion to the back and neck. To lessen the strain, a chair with armrests can be used to help support our elbows as we hold the book up, or you can lean your wrists on a table in front of you while holding a book or paper. Alternatively a writing slope is a great way of supporting your book on a desk or table, so that it is tilted toward you.

A writing slope tilts the paper or book towards you.

Exercise – Sitting reading

- Sit far back in an upright chair with armrests. Your feet should be on the floor and your back supported by a chair-back or firm cushion.
- 'Inhibit' picking up the book, but attend to your poise first.
- Free your neck by letting your head nod forward a few millimetres on the top vertebra. Think of your head going upward and your back lengthening and widening.
- Now, reach for your book while avoiding stiffening your neck. Move with thought and care.
- Hold the book in two hands and rest your elbows on the armrests.
- Allow your head to roll forward a little on the very top joint of your spine without dropping your entire neck forward. You can look downward with your eyes.
- Free your neck again and think upward with your head while reading.
- If you are sitting on a chair without arms, bring yourself upright by directing as described above and raise your book up toward you. Bear in mind that your arms and the book are of a considerable weight, so you can allow your body to lean backward by just a few degrees to compensate, so your overall body weight remains in balance.
- Do not get stuck leaning forward as you will put excessive weight into your hip joints, causing your sacrum, legs and abdomen to stiffen. Lean forward and backward occasionally to vary your poise and avoid strain.

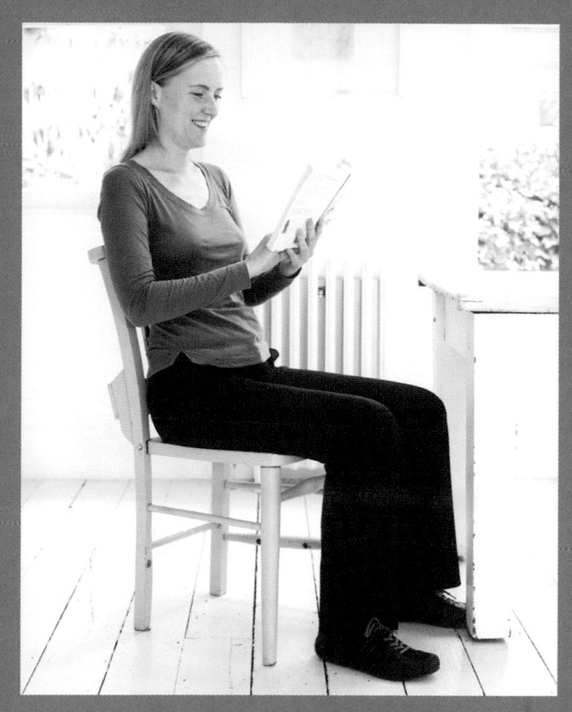

Put your bottom to the back of the chair and use the chair back for support.

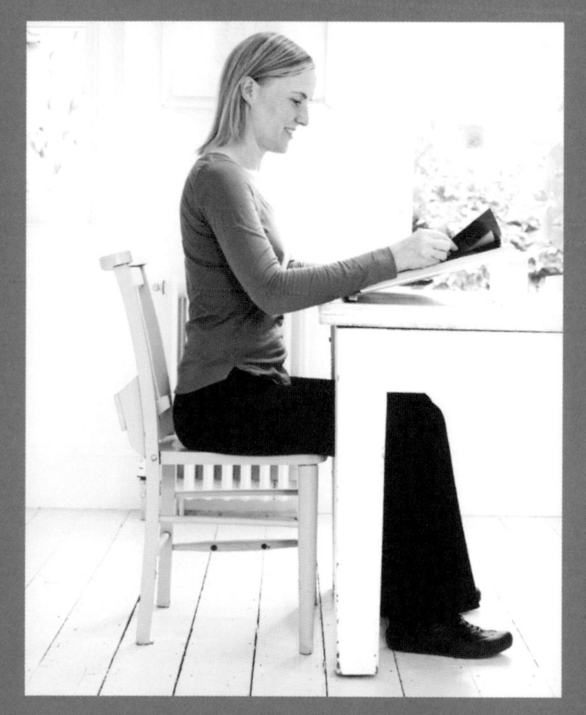

Keep your distance from the book. Do not get drawn down towards it.

Sitting on a sofa or soft chair

The same principles apply to sitting on a soft chair. The main difference is that we do not get the same sense of our sitting bones being supported as they sink downward and the soft cushions behind us tend to give way. This means we have nowhere to lengthen up from. Invariably we end up collapsed in stature and slouched.

Try to position a firm cushion behind you so you can at least feel supported in your back. Let your feet rest flat on the floor in front of you, or if you are sitting too far back to do so, raise your legs on a stool so you are more reclined. Free your neck and release your shoulders.

Use cushions for support and free your neck.

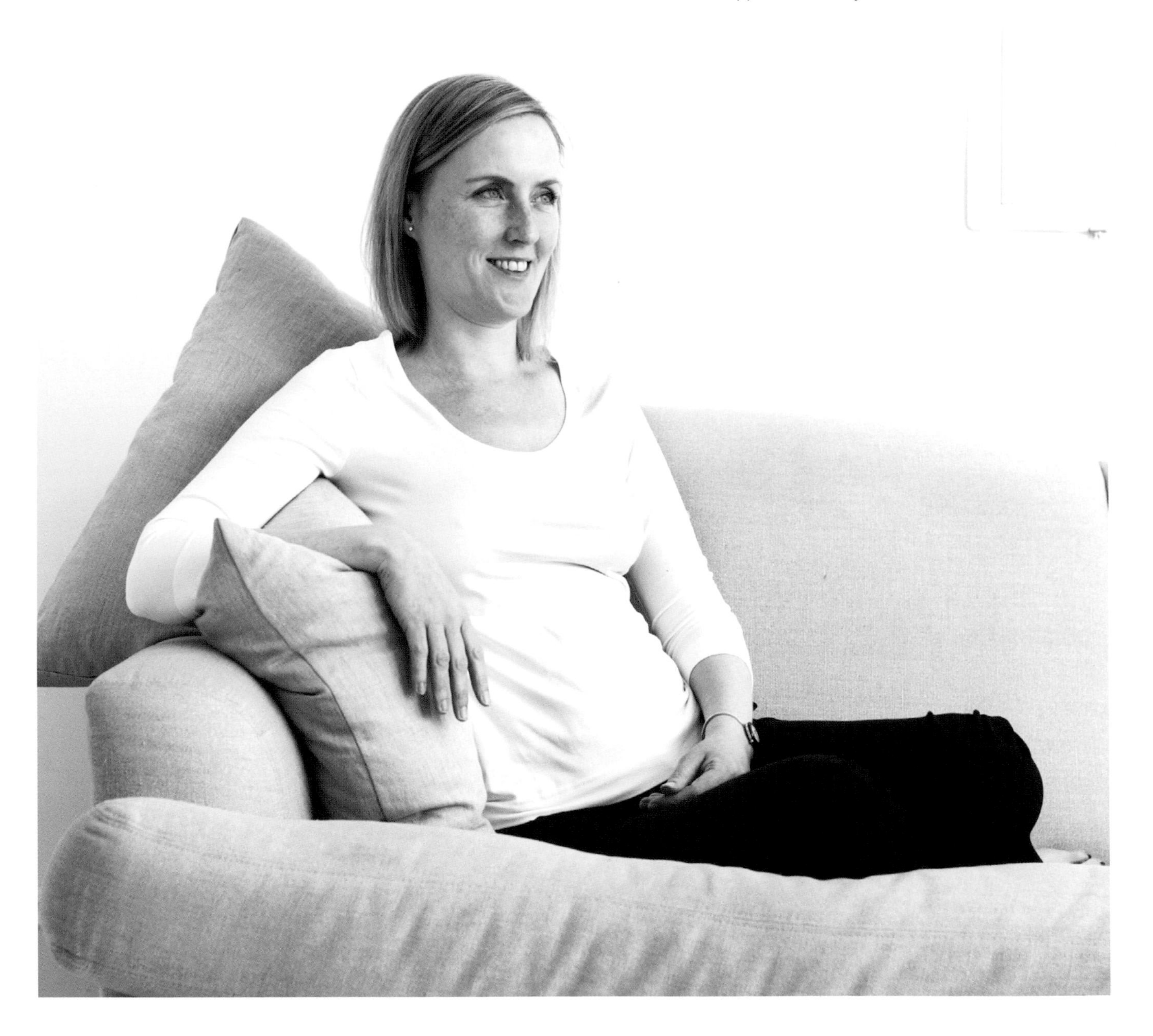

Sitting at a dining table

Chairs are rarely ideal so we need to look after ourselves, rather than relying on chair design. Balance is key for avoiding strain, so sense your sitting bones underneath you and give your directions to help maintain upright poise. Free your neck, 'direct' your head upward and think of lengthening and widening. Use the back of the chair for support if it's reasonable.

However it's important not to get stuck. So vary how you sit to avoid strain or tension creeping in.

HELPFUL TIPS

›› Position yourself to the back of the chair and use the chair-back to support you when resting.

›› To eat, you may bring yourself forward in the chair. Balance on your sitting bones and free your neck.

›› To lean forward, do so by moving from your hips as in the exercise, 'Leaning forward when sitting' (page 119).

›› Keep your feet flat on the floor. Avoid wrapping them around each other or around the legs of the chair.

›› Don't sit in a twist but square on to the table.

›› Avoid leaning on the table with one elbow and eating with just a fork as this puts you in a twist. Either place one hand on your lap as you eat with a fork, or use both knife and fork.

A free neck and expansive poise helps us be relaxed, confident and pain free.

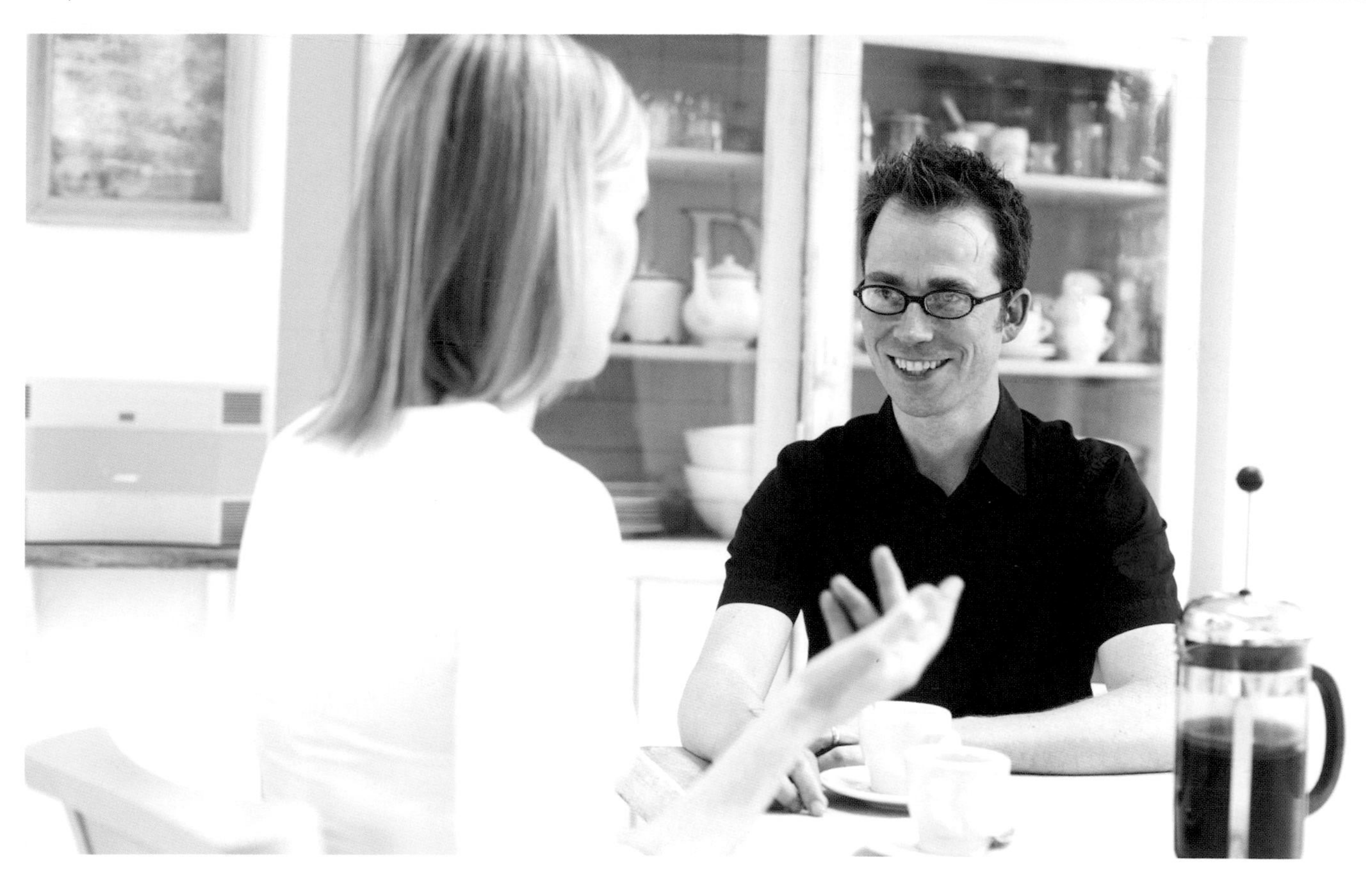

Sitting at a computer

There are inherent difficulties of sitting at a computer such as being drawn forward to peer at the screen and hunching over the keyboard. As with all sitting situations, we need to be in good balance to avoid unnecessary strain in the back, neck and shoulders. Sitting too long in front of a computer slouched or stiff is sure to bring on back pain, so we must learn to look after ourselves in the process.

Many companies are very conscious of providing healthy working conditions for their employees and may even offer the services of an ergonomic specialist to sort out your work station so it is most appropriate for your height and needs. However, no matter how well your desk and chair are set up, you must still avoid habitually tensing or slouching. If you are to avoid back pain, good balance is essential and you need to be lengthening and widening in stature.

HELPFUL TIPS

›› Adjust your chair height so your elbows are level or above your wrists when typing.

›› Adjust the chair armrests so they support your elbow without you needing to raise or drop your shoulders.

›› Feet should be flat on the floor or on a foot-rest without stretching. Always ensure your feet are supported.

›› Sit back in the chair, sense your sitting bones under you. Now adjust the lumbar back of the chair to support a gentle lumbar curve. It should neither push your back in nor collapse your back outward. Do not overdo it! Less is better than more.

›› Avoid having the chair-back leaning backward as this will cause you to drop your head and neck forward. Bring the chair-back upright.

›› Position the screen so that it is in front of you and your keyboard below. The screen should not be so high as to cause you to tilt your head backward. You should be able to glance from screen to keys by only using your eyes.

›› Free your neck and let your head roll forward a little on top of your spine.

›› Type lightly with as little effort as possible. Avoid arching your wrists and flattening your hands. Your hands should be gently curved so little pressure is used by your fingers to type.

›› Take frequent breaks. Get up every 30 minutes to move around, get a glass of water.

›› Don't get stuck in one position.

›› Breathe.

Sit on your sitting bones, free your neck and keep your distance from the screen.

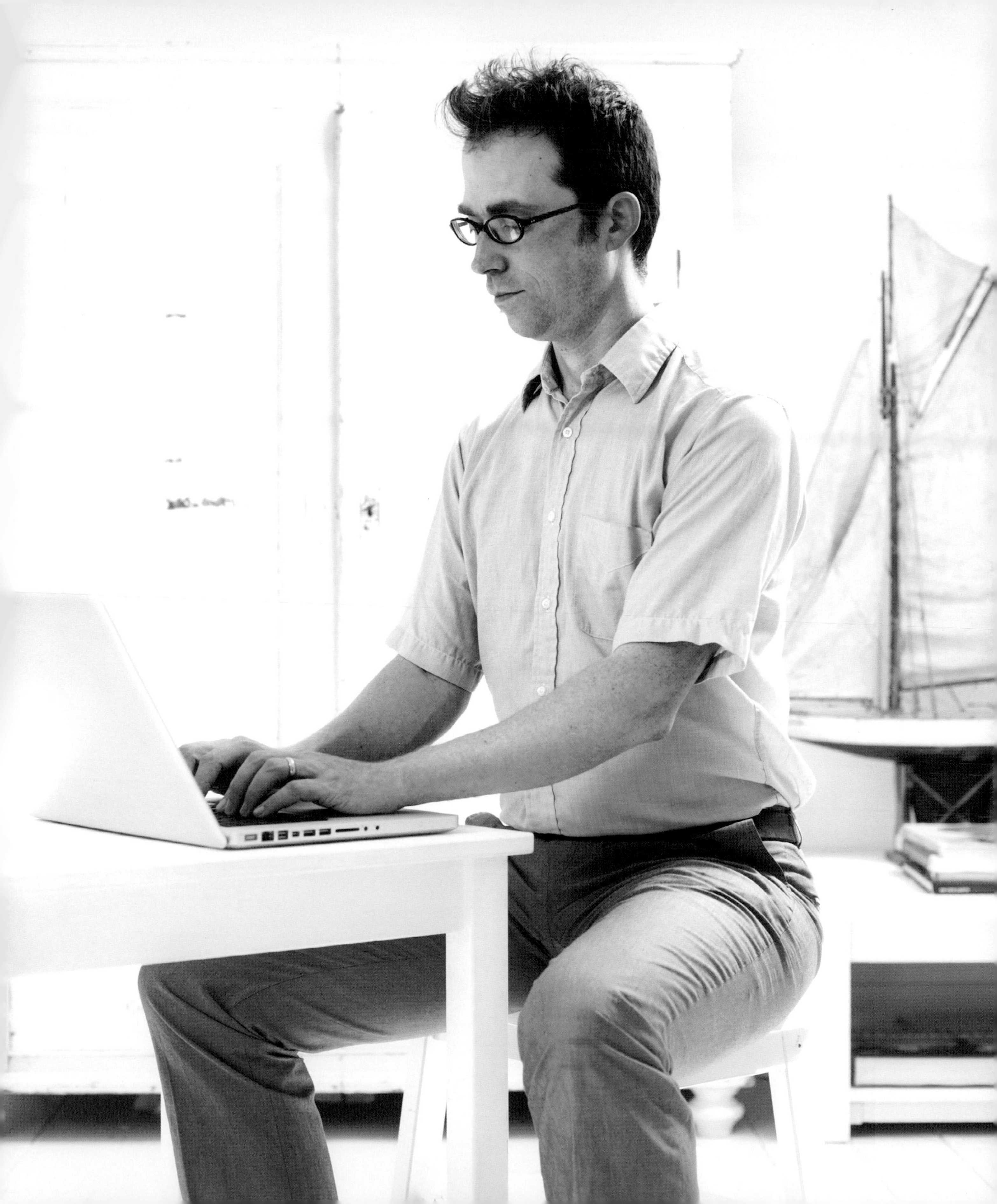

Driving

Car seats are renowned for being uncomfortable and can contribute to causing back pain during long journeys. They may be designed for an average person, but who is average? We need to make the most of the situation to avoid lumbar pain or a stiff neck and shoulders.

Most car seats are too soft to offer proper support, particularly in old cars. Experiment with using a hard foam seat wedge or lumbar cushion. Be aware of how you are sitting and use the Alexander Technique to help you by inhibiting and directing.

HELPFUL TIPS

- Always sit back against the chair-back.
- Gently adjust the lumbar support if it has one, or position a flat cushion or folded scarf behind your lumbar back.
- Avoid leaning your head back against the head rest; it is really only there to prevent whiplash in an emergency.
- Bring your seat into a fairly upright position so that you are not over-reaching for the steering wheel when your hands are at 'ten-to-two' with elbows gently bent.
- Slide the seat forward so you are not stretching to reach the pedals.
- 'Direct' your neck to be free and your head to go forward and upward, back to lengthen and widen, knees forward and away.
- Adjust your rear-view mirror so you can see easily without changing your position.
- Don't grip the wheel. Allow your neck and shoulders to release and lightly hold the steering wheel. Have a sense of your arms connecting to your mid-back. Relax your fingers.
- Don't let your left foot hover over the clutch pedal. Rest it flat on the floor until needed.
- Remember to breathe and stop often for a rest.

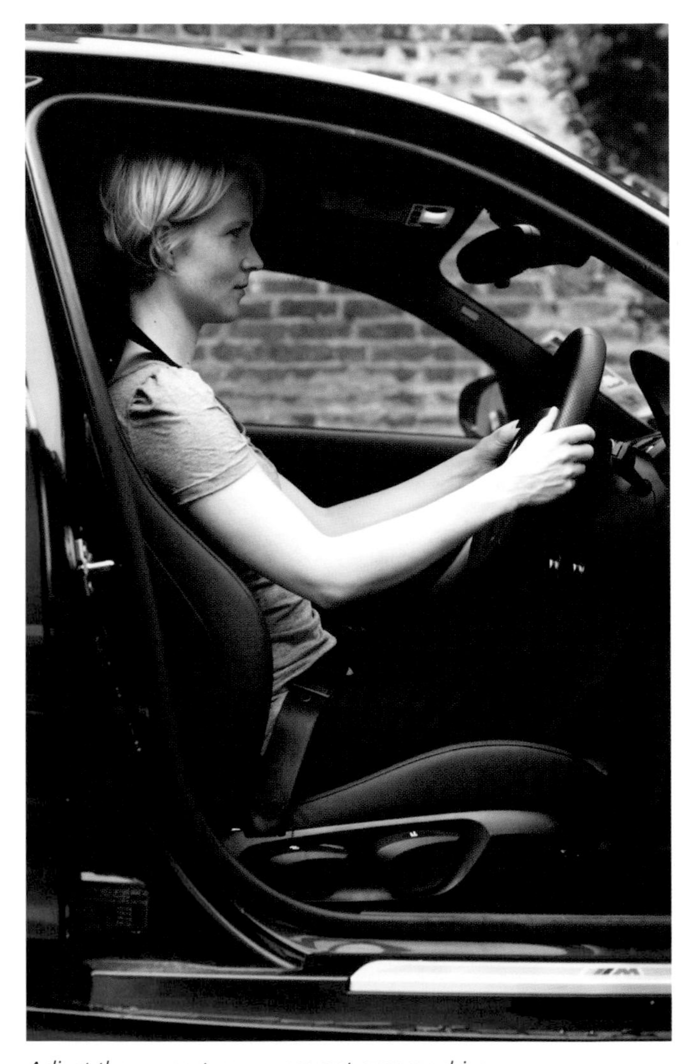

Adjust the car seat so you are not over-reaching.

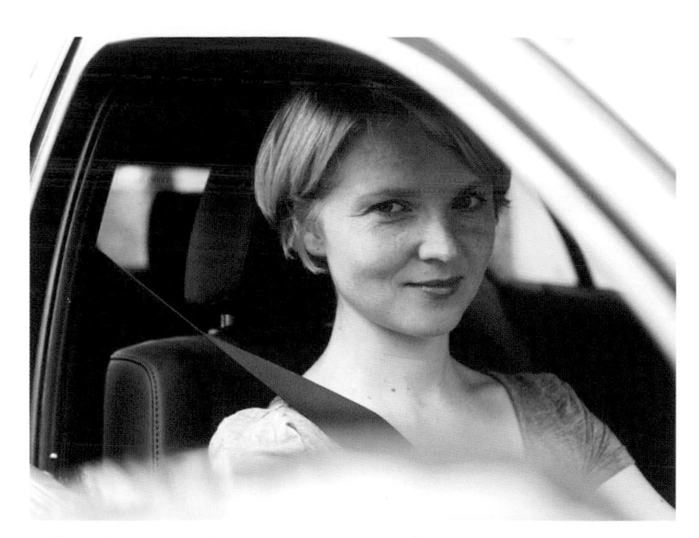

Adjust the wing mirror so you can simply turn your eyes.

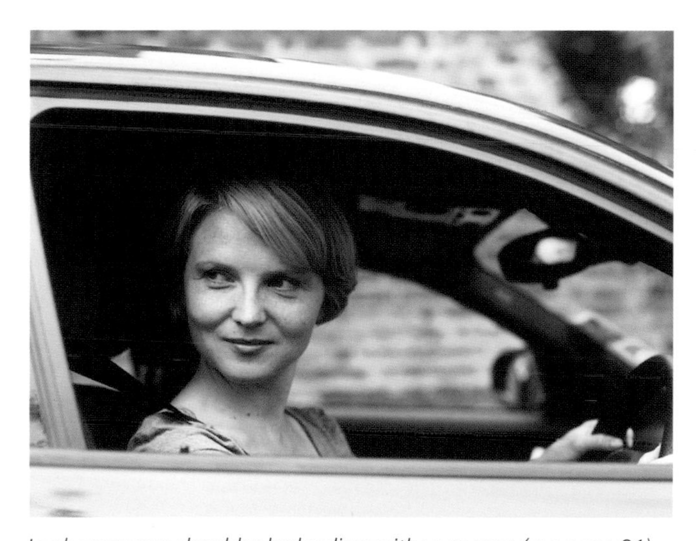

Look over your shoulder by leading with your eyes (see page 91).

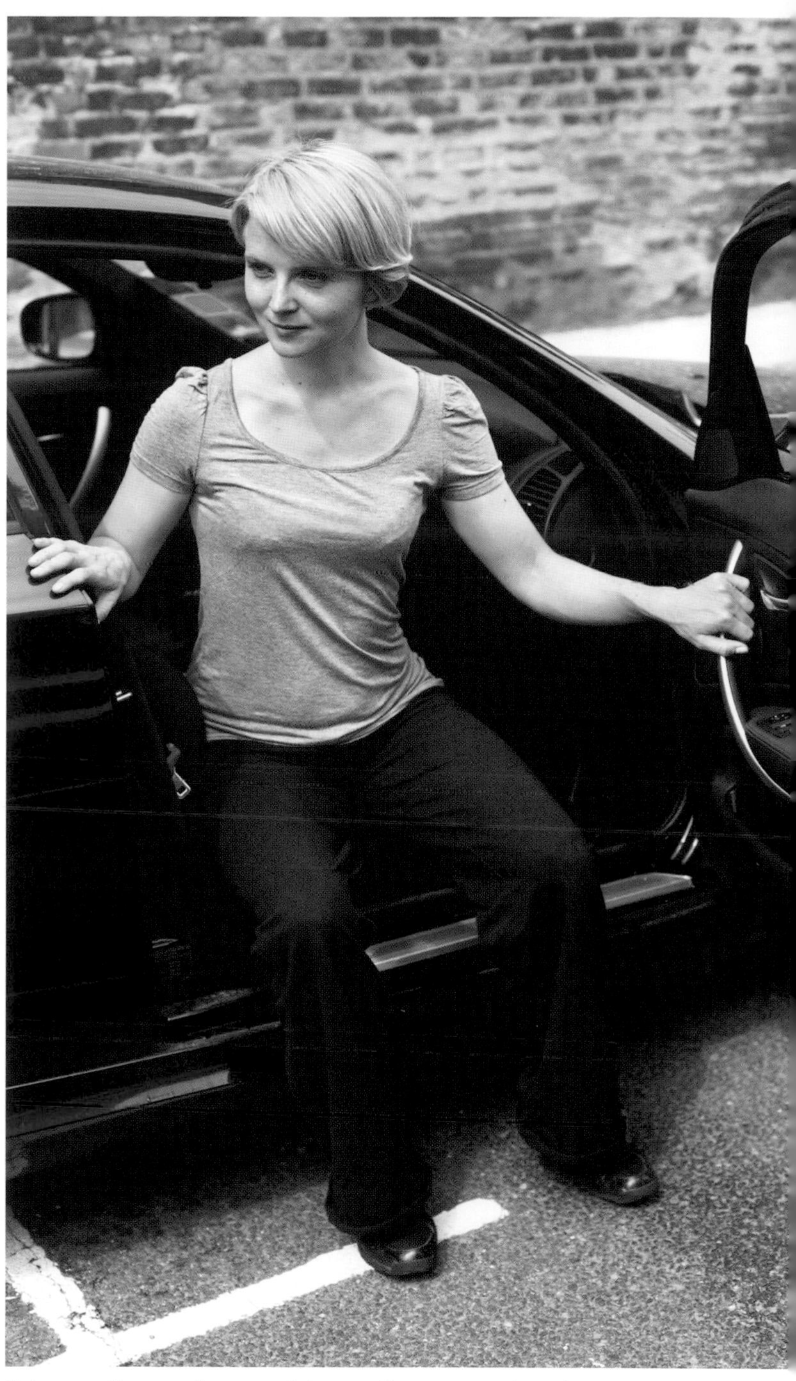

Take your time getting out of the car. Free your neck and direct upward.

Walking

We will enjoy healthy pain-free walking when we are expansive in stature, moving lightly in good balance with a free neck. We will then expend the minimum of energy and avoid discomfort.

As young children, we walk effortlessly until we develop postural habits that interfere with our muscle co-ordination. As soon as we become stooped or slouched and lose the quality of expansiveness we experience pain and waste huge amounts of energy.

Thankfully we have the musculature to allow easy walking without strain. We just need to re-learn it and the Alexander Technique will help us.

When we stoop and slouch we collapse and disengage all the supportive muscles that are intended to carry us around. Consequently we end up stiffening to compensate for the lack of support while also trying harder than necessary to move. If we 'go up' as Alexander would have said, we activate the musculature to support us better and we can move with a lightness of foot.

In cities and towns where the majority of us spend our time, we walk on even floors, pavements and roads that have no variation in levels, angles or roughness of ground. They are all very flat and consequently our feet fall with exactly the same movement and alignment with every step. This leads to a very repetitive walking pattern that can cause wear and tear on our feet, knees and hips, not to mention our back. Uneven ground, however, constantly changes our step and balance so there is more variety of movement and less wear on specific joints; a far healthier environment. Living in cities and towns means we need to take even more care in how we walk as the repetitive pattern of walking is unremitting and can cause rapid deterioration and physical disabilities.

Let's look at walking in more detail.

The main requirement for healthy pain-free walking is an ability to stand evenly on two feet and be in good balance while also lengthening and widening in stature. We achieve this quality by means of Alexander's method and it applies to walking as much as sitting, standing or bending.

Walking can be considered as simply moving one foot in front of another then transferring our body weight onto each foot in turn. However with some care and attention we can help ourselves walk freely and avoid harmful habits from interfering such as shortening and getting off balance. The key is that we need to release unnecessary tension and to lengthen in stature with every stride. This is how we have evolved as a species to walk, and this is how we need to do it now; there are no exceptions that won't cause harmful deterioration and pain. It is how we are made.

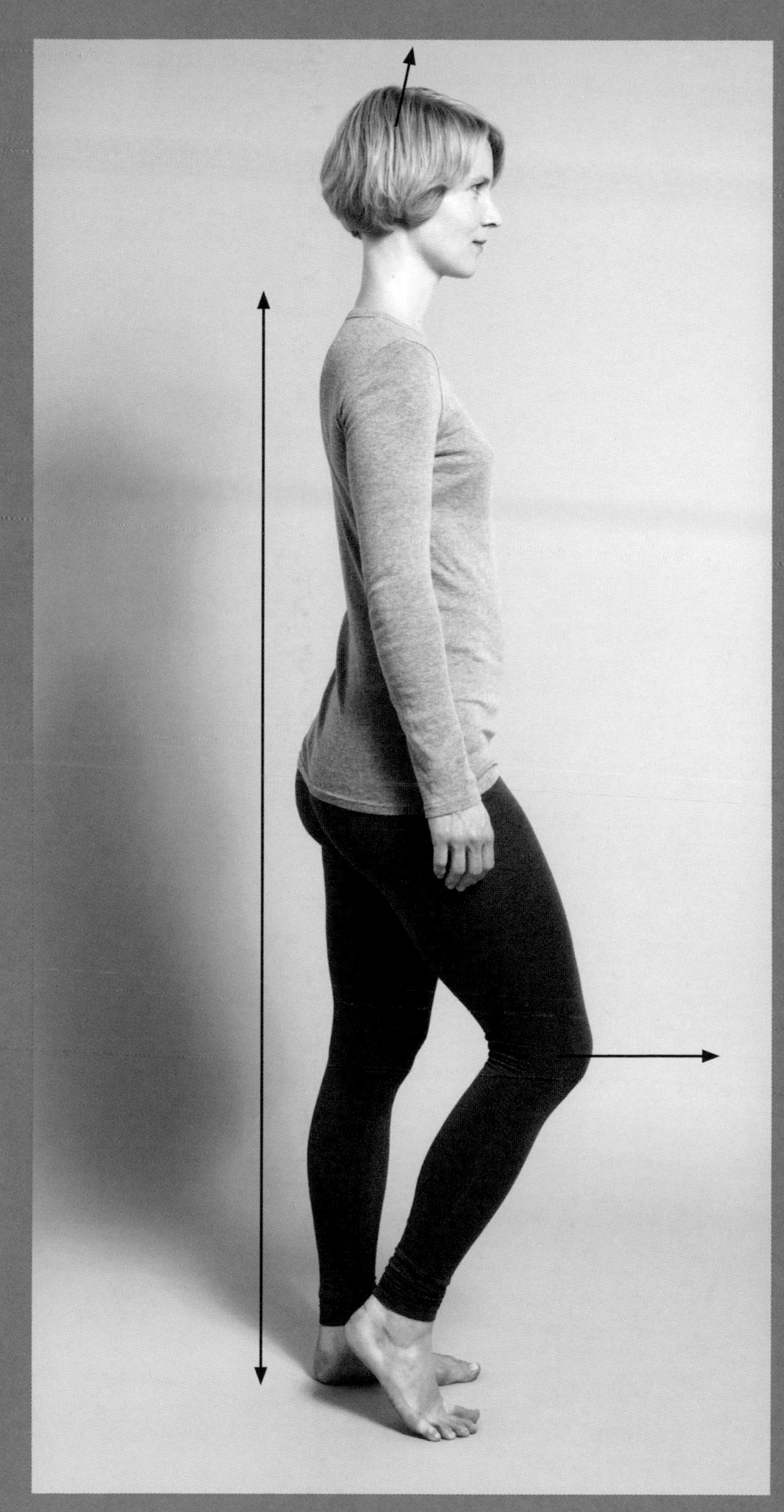

Free your neck, direct your head upward and lead the leg movement with your knee

Exercise – Preparing to walk

This exercise is like walking on the spot. Practise without lifting your toes off the floor.

›› Stand evenly on both feet, spaced 7–10cm (3–4 inches) apart.

›› 'Inhibit' doing anything and give time to think.

›› Free your neck by letting your head roll forward on the top of your spine, 'direct' your head to go forward and upward, your back to lengthen and widen. 'Inhibit' straining or pushing.

›› In a moment you will bend one knee forward over your big toe. But you will do so by giving the correct 'direction' to activate the musculature. You must 'direct' (think) your head upward to lengthen in your back in order to bend your knee. It is the lengthening of your back (led by your head) that brings about the correct co-ordination to do it easily and lightly.

›› 'Direct' your neck to be free and send your head upward, then bend one knee forward so it is pointing. Keep your toes on the floor. Now return your heel to the floor and let your leg straighten, but think your head upward again.

›› Repeat with the other knee.

›› Avoid collapsing the opposite hip. Do not sway.

›› Repeat slowly for 30–60 seconds.

›› Rest.

›› Do the exercise again. First 'inhibit' and give yourself time to think.

Exercise – Walking

This exercise is exactly the same as before, but you will now put one foot out in front of the other.

- First 'inhibit' rushing to give yourself time to think.
- Establish your free, upright poise by inhibiting and directing as above.
- Free your neck, 'direct' your head forward and upward to lengthen in your back as you bend one knee forward and away. Let your foot go a short step forward and place your heel on the floor in front of you.
- Let your head roll forward on top of your spine before moving your whole body weight over your front foot. Your head must go upward, over the front foot to lead the way.
- As you move forward, allow your rear knee to bend. Think upward with your head as you move your knee forward so your foot comes through and the heel lands a short step in front of you.
- Lead each step with your knee, not your foot.
- Avoid swaying from side to side. You can keep a straight line if you 'direct' your head upward as you walk. Look ahead of you.

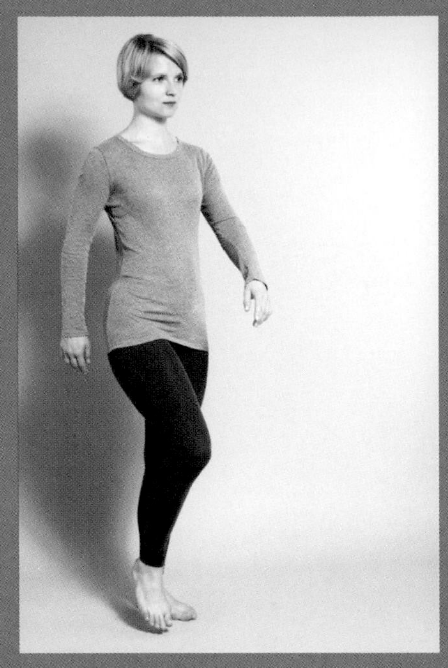

1. Direct your head upward and lead with your knee.

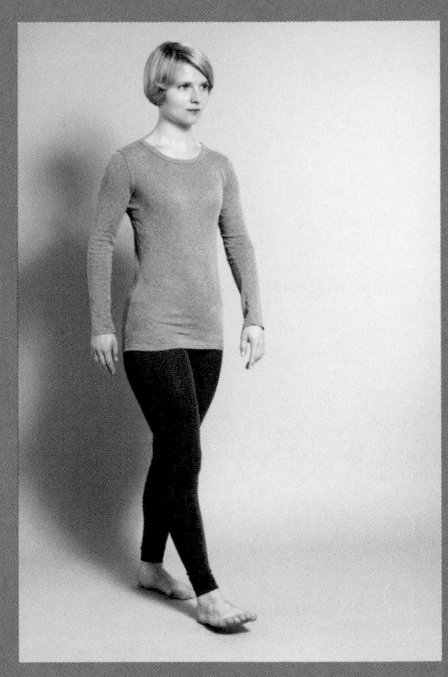

2. Keep your weight back so you are not leaning.

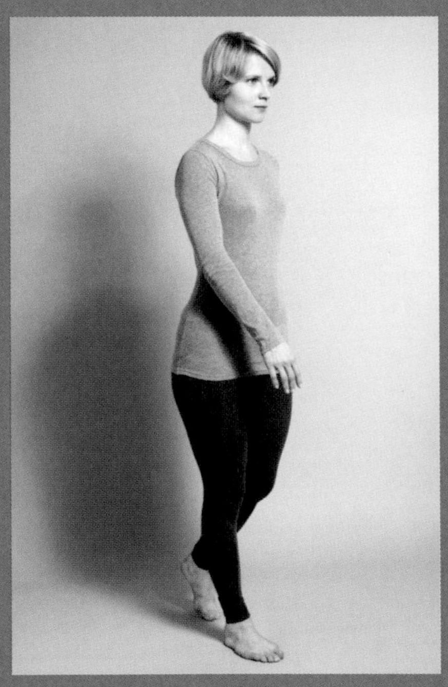

3. Let your head roll forward as you move over the front foot.

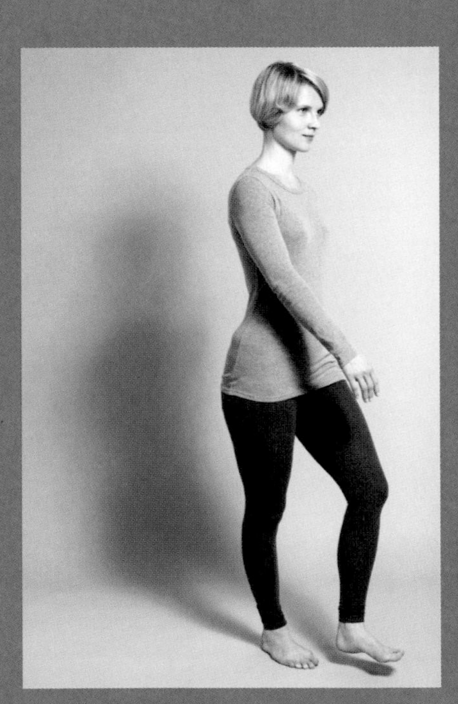

4. Lengthen with every step.

HELPFUL TIPS

›› Free your neck and 'direct' your head upward.

›› Take short strides rather than long.

›› Avoid arching your back or pushing your hips forward.

›› Send your bending knees over your toes, so the knee does not come inward. Directing your knees forward and away helps to release your hips and lower back.

›› Keep your weight back so you are not leaning forward.

›› Allow your arms to swing freely at your sides. The arm opposite to your bending knee should swing forward and help your walking rhythm.

›› Avoid swaying from side to side. 'Direct' your head upward to stabilise your body.

›› Walk as freely as possible. Make less effort.

›› To avoid plodding, think upward with your head. Think of walking lightly.

›› Carry as little as possible. Wear a back pack or a shoulder bag diagonally. If you carry a shoulder or hand bag, change sides often.

›› Avoid looking at the ground other than to glance for safety reasons. Look ahead to where you are walking and take in your surroundings. It will help you lengthen.

›› Sit down often.

Footwear

Consideration should be given to the shoes you wear as they can make quite a difference in your manner of walking and help avoid backache. Shoes should ideally give proper support to your feet and have a low heel. High heels tend to throw your weight forward causing you to compensate by arching your back. They can also cause shortening of your hamstrings which make it difficult to bend while also encouraging your foot to slide forward in the shoe, causing pinching of toes and possible bunions.

Orthotic inserts may be recommended by some podiatrists and they can provide more support to your feet and possibly alleviate back pain. But bear in mind that orthotics act as a crutch to support the arch of your feet – a job that should be done by the muscles of your legs – and by so doing encourage a weakening of leg muscle which can make your legs and feet work even less efficiently. It is my belief that they should only be used in difficult circumstances and it is far better to re-train your leg muscles to support you by means of using the Alexander Technique that restores natural poise.

Climbing stairs

Walking up stairs is not much different from walking on the flat. If our tendency is to stoop and shorten in stature when climbing stairs, we are effectively 'coming down' on ourselves when our legs are going up, compressing our back and all our joints. We should 'direct' our head forward and upward so we lengthen as we climb the stairs. This will make us move more lightly and avoid plodding.

HELPFUL TIPS

›› Look ahead when climbing stairs. Do not look down as it will cause you to plod.

›› Keep your weight back on the rear foot. Avoid leaning on the front foot. Think of 'going up' off your rear foot.

›› Lengthen in stature with each step.

›› Think of your head 'floating' up ahead of you.

Exercise – Climbing stairs

›› Stand at the foot of the stairs with your feet parallel.

›› 'Inhibit' doing anything to give time to think and use the 'means-whereby' approach.

›› Free your neck and 'direct' your head forward and upward, back to lengthen and widen.

›› Move your right knee forward and upward so your foot comes onto the first step.

›› Pause. Keep your weight on the back foot. Don't lean.

›› Release your neck. 'Direct' your head forward and upward away from your back foot and allow your body weight to transfer onto the right foot.

›› 'Direct' your head forward and upward to initiate the movement of your left knee so your foot comes up onto the next step.

›› Lead with your head to initiate the movement of your right knee forward and up, so your foot arrives on the next step.

›› For every step, direct upwards to initiate the movement of your knee.

›› Repeat.

Note: Keep your weight back on the rear foot and 'direct' your head upward to avoid plodding.

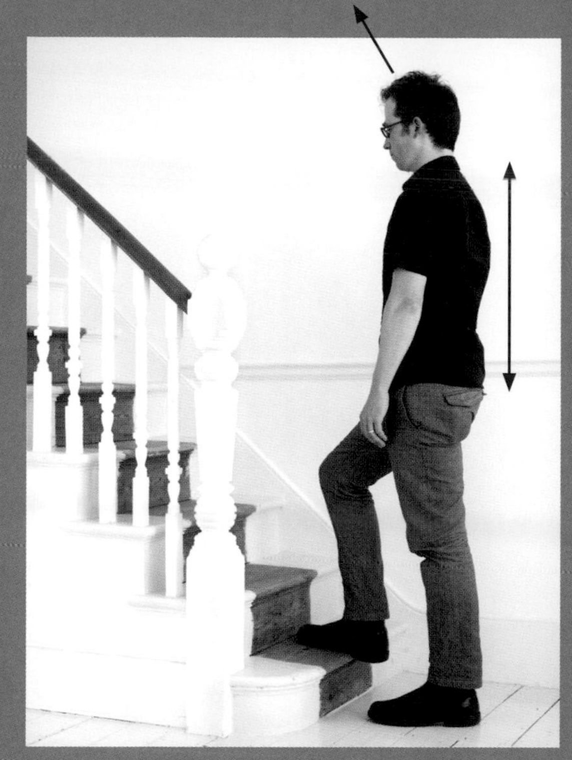

1. Direct your head upward and lead with your knee.

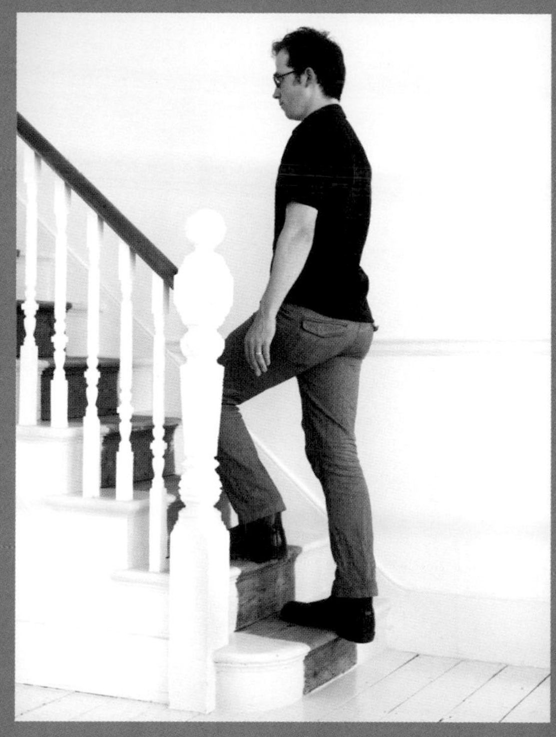

2. Keep your weight back and think upward.

When walking down stairs, again free your neck and send your head upward! There is no reason to shorten in stature as you go down stairs. You still want the best co-ordination of muscles and they work at their optimum if you are lengthening in stature. Glance down occasionally but send your head upward and lengthen in the front of your body. Do so and you'll feel wonderfully light. Use a hand rail for safety if you are feeling insecure at not looking down.

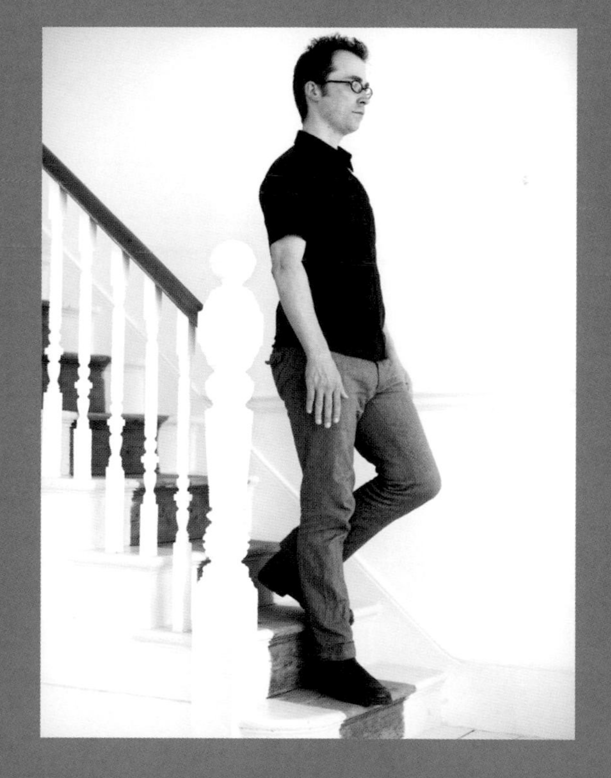

3. Lengthen in stature as you descend.

Bending

The need to bend presents itself many times a day and can be a real cause for concern if we have a painful back. Indeed bending can be the 'final straw' if we have postural problems and can trigger a muscle spasm or trapped nerve. But if we bend with care, there is no reason why we cannot do so without pain and avoid problems in the future. It is worthwhile experimenting to change how you bend.

The key to bending healthily to avoid problems is to always be in balance. This not only involves bending at our knees, but also bending freely in all our joints so no interference prevents us from moving smoothly. We also want to expend the least amount of energy. So bending should not be seen as an activity of our legs, but involving the whole of our body from our head down. As the saying goes, 'Many hands make light work'; utilising a great many muscles means we can 'make light work' of bending. Make bending a 'lengthening activity', not a 'shortening activity'.

HELPFUL TIPS

- Spread your feet apart for stability, possibly one foot in advance of the other.
- Get as close to the item as possible.
- Breathe out as you bend.
- Check the weight of the item gently.
- Come back on your ankles so your whole body weight adjusts to accommodate the weight of the object being lifted.
- To return to standing, 'inhibit' to free your neck. Send your head upward to lead the way to standing.

Exercise – Bending

Note: Don't 'end-gain'. 'Inhibit' rushing ahead so you can use a 'means-whereby' approach. Think.

- This exercise is very similar to Monkey Position.
- Stand with your feet further apart than usual – about 45cm (18in). Turn your feet outward slightly.
- Pause. 'Inhibit'. Give yourself time to think. Bring your weight back over your ankles.
- Do not think of 'going down'. Free your neck, 'direct' your head forward and upward, lengthen and widen in your back.
- When you bend, you will free your neck again first by letting your head nod forward a few millimetres.
- Allow your knees to bend 'forward and away' over your toes. At the same time, bend forward at your hips, i.e. your bottom goes backward and your knees go forward.
- The degree of the bend of your knees and hips should be roughly similar.
- Now you are in 'Monkey'. Allow your arms to hang freely at your sides.
- To pick something up, bend further so you can take hold of the object.
- To return to standing, pause. 'Inhibit' to give yourself time to bring your body weight back and redistribute it evenly over your ankles, given that you may now have a weighty item in your hands. Free your neck and 'direct' your head upward so you return to standing.

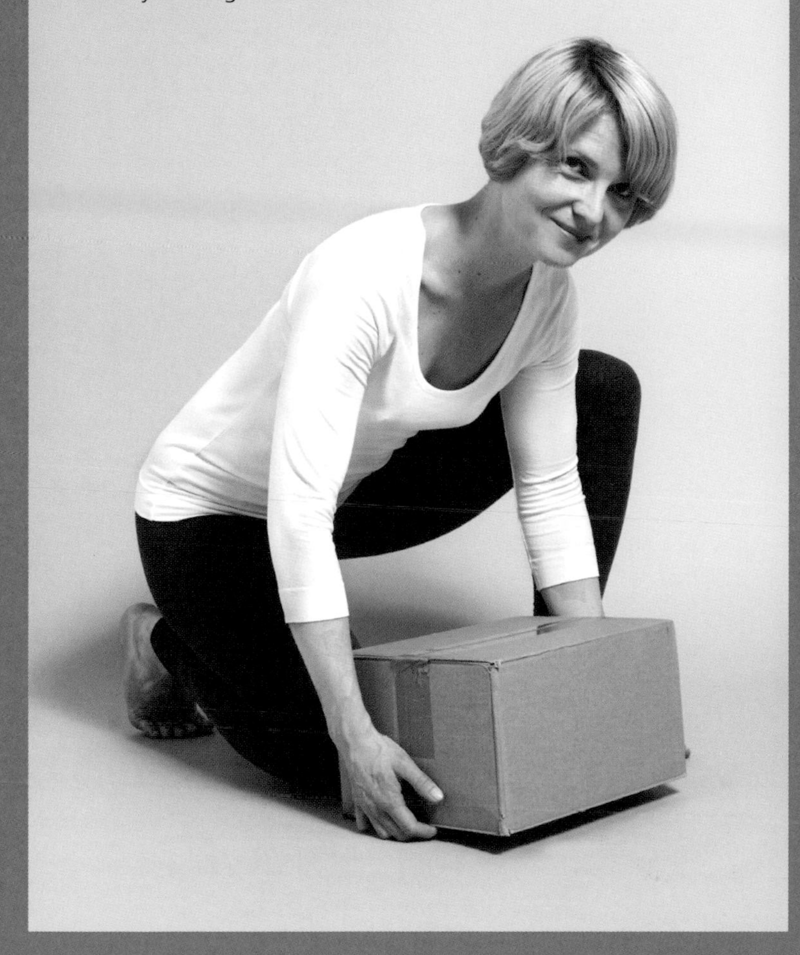

1. Free your neck and direct upward.
Keep the weight close.

2. Bend through Monkey Position.

3. When lifting heavy objects, position your weight over the item.

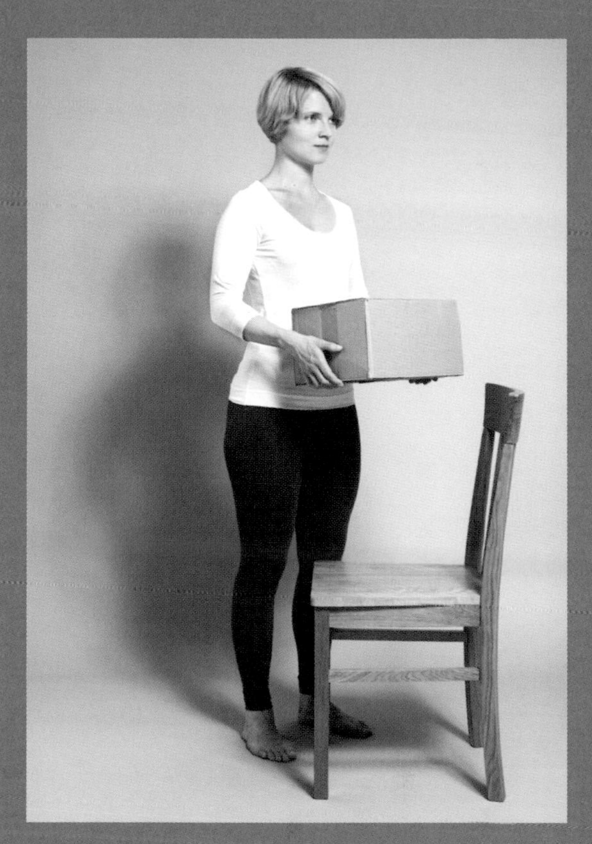

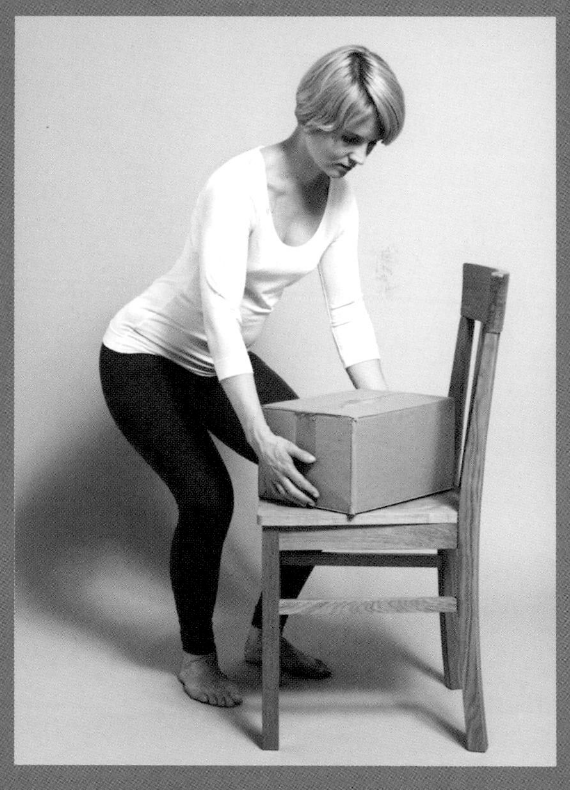

Bending in this way utilises your whole body so no one part is taking the strain.

You can do the same exercise by placing one foot slightly in advance of the other in a mini-lunge position. This offers more stability and you can go down on one knee.

Carrying

Carrying things is a necessity of life and we should be mindful of how we do so, to avoid straining our back. Bear in mind that any item adds weight to our body, consequently there is going to be a strain unless we are in good balance. Being in good balance when carrying something means adapting to the situation so our body can compensate for the extra weight.

You need your back to be lengthening and widening as this provides the best support, enables more efficient use of your legs and arms and also involves less effort.

Exercise – Adapting your balance to cope with carrying a weight

This exercise lets you experiment with adjusting your balance with a weight.

›› Place a pile of books on a table and stand close.

›› 'Inhibit' doing anything. Establish good balance over your ankles. Avoid leaning.

›› Free your neck, 'direct' your head forward and upward, lengthen and widen in your back.

›› You are now going to pick up the pile of books.

›› 'Inhibit'. Let your head nod forward as you reach out to pick up the books.

›› Lead with your head as you come up to your full height.

›› Hold the pile of books close to your body. Free your ankles so you are evenly balanced.

›› In a moment, you will stretch your arms out straight in front of you, holding the books. When you do so, free your neck by letting your head roll forward a few millimetres.

›› When you hold the pile of books away from your body, allow your whole weight to move backward from your ankles to compensate for the weight in front. Avoid arching your back.

›› Bring the books back toward your body. Notice how your weight sways forward to upright.

›› Hold the books away from you again and notice how you automatically lean back from your ankles to compensate.

›› Bring the books back to your body. Pause before putting them down on the table. Free your neck, bend your knees, hips and ankles if you bend down.

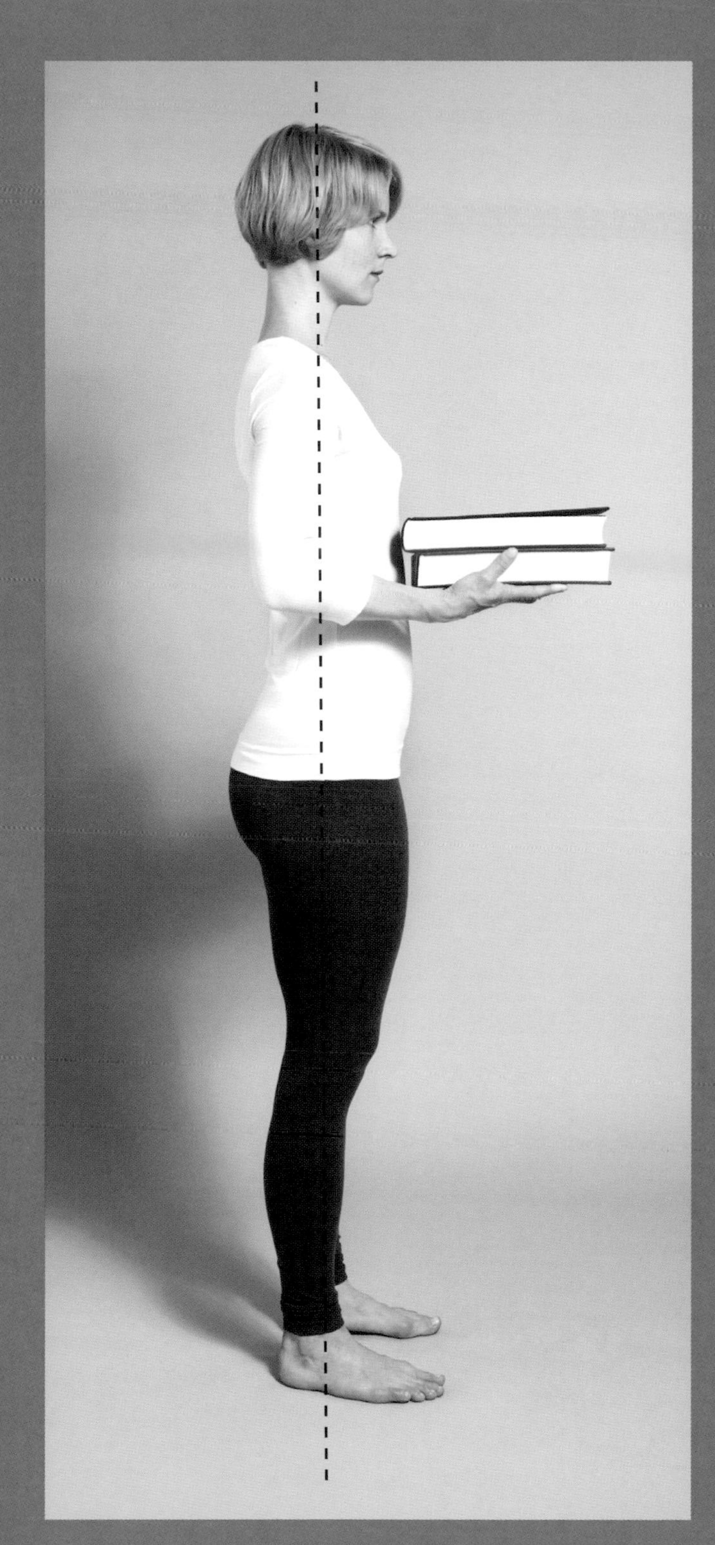

Standing in balance, books close to your body.

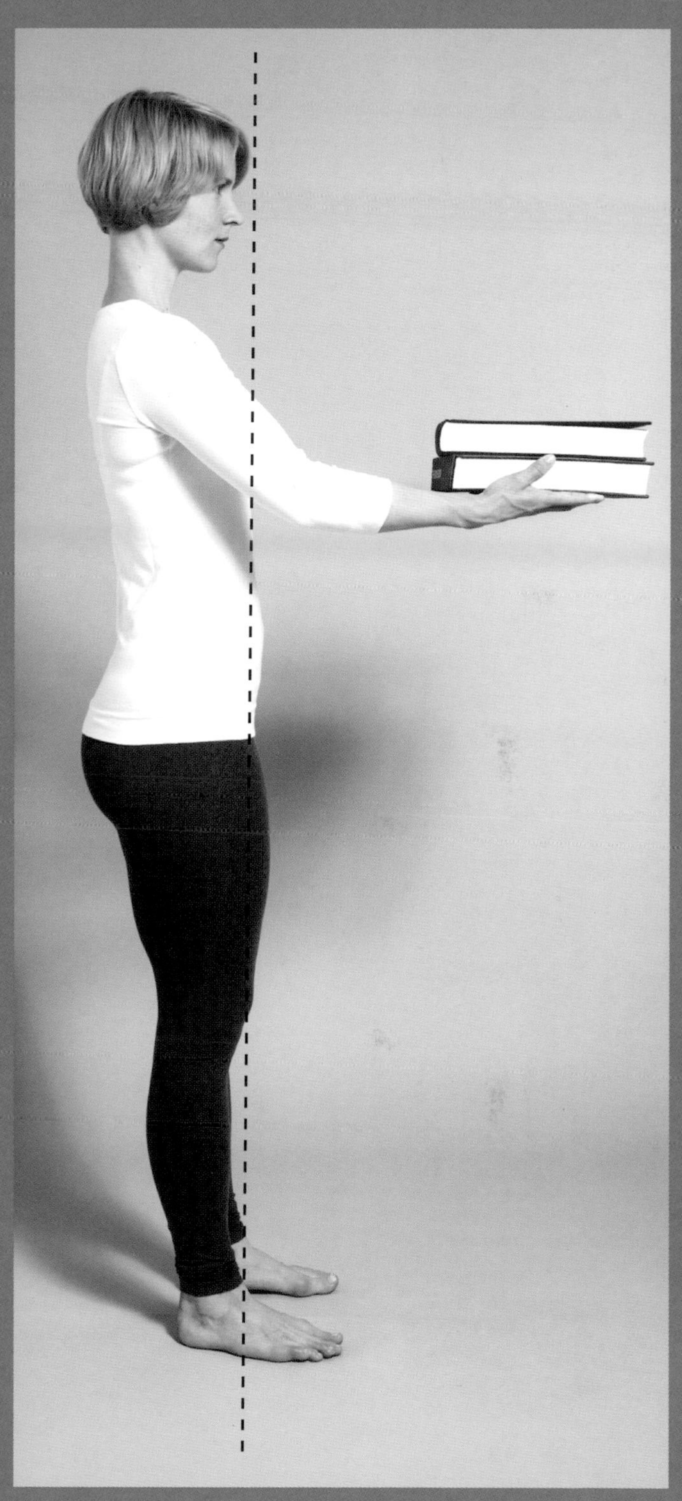

Hold the books away and allow yourself to come backwards from the ankles. Avoid arching your back.

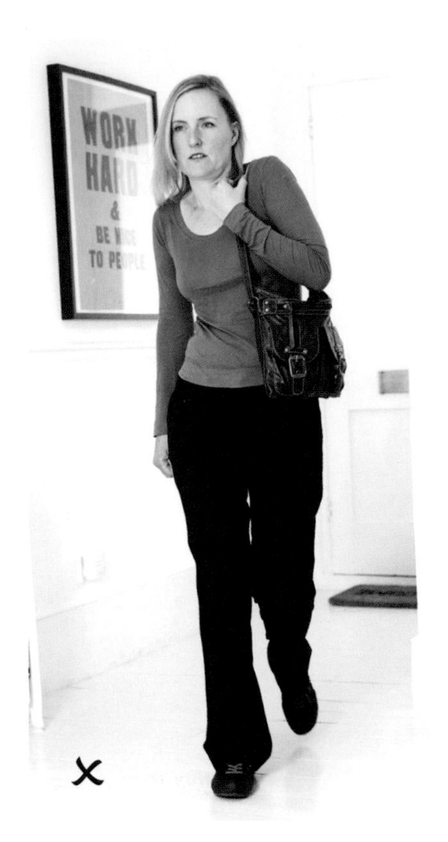

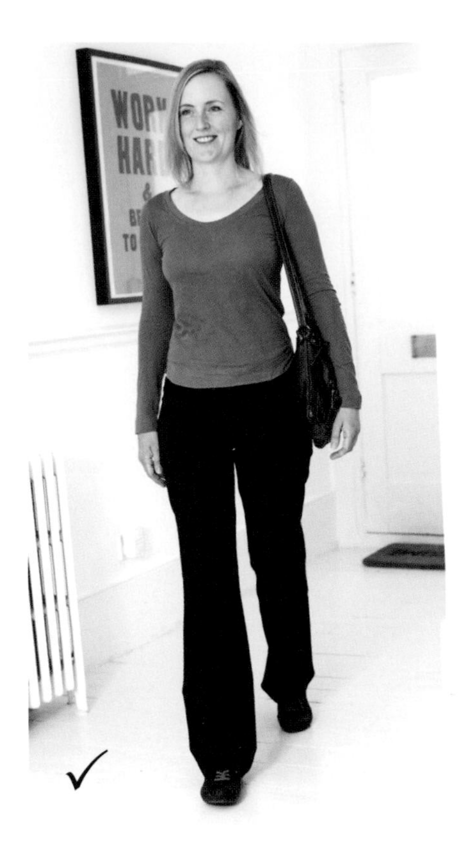

l. *Hunched shoulder, stiff neck and twisted.*

r. *Walking freely, lengthening in stature.*

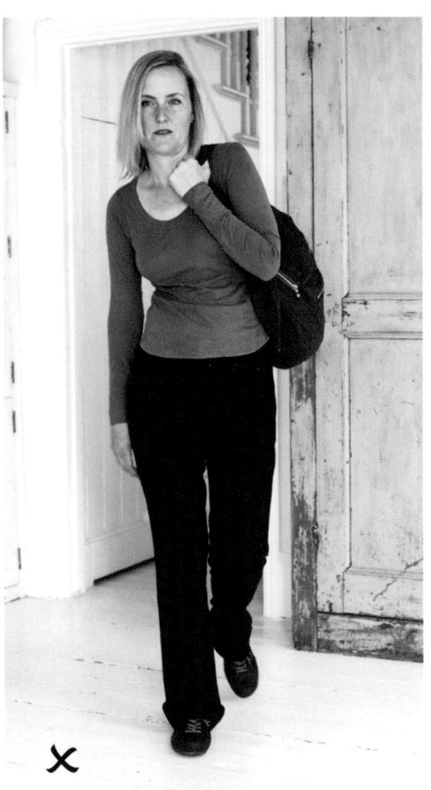

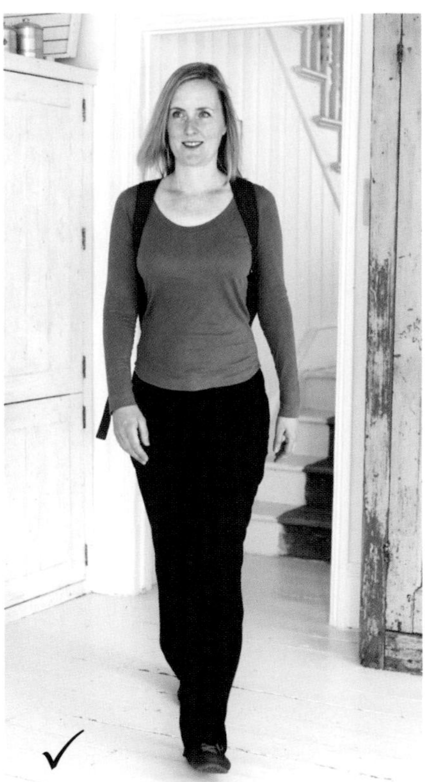

l. *A backpack worn on one shoulder causes you to twist.*

r. *Wear the backpack with both straps for even weight distribution.*

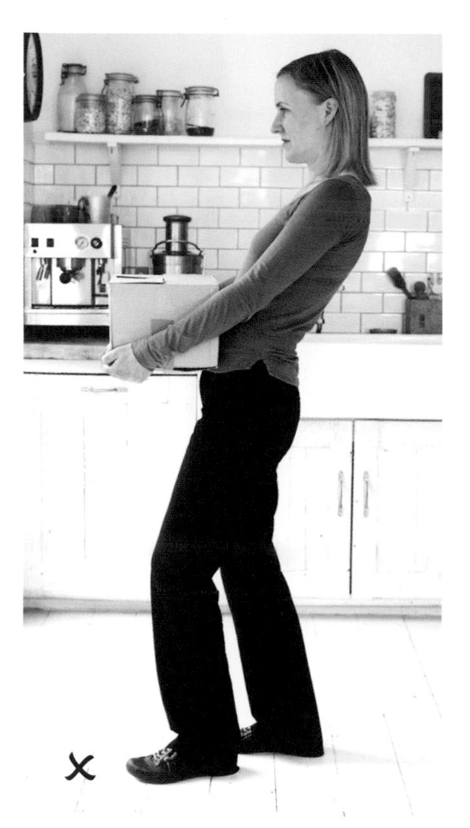

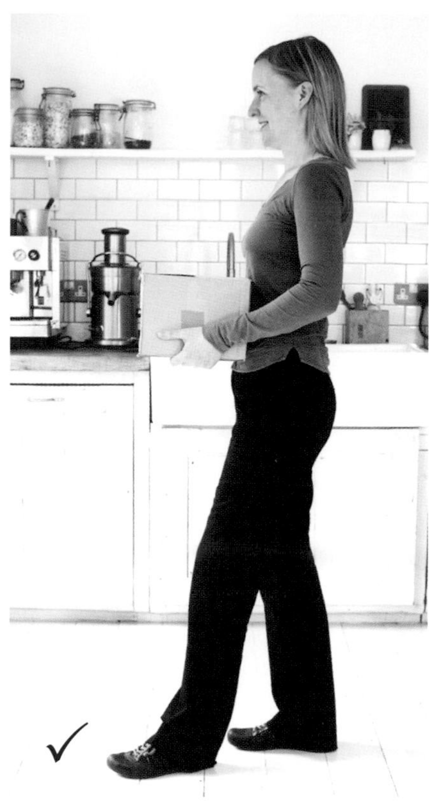

l. *Arching your back causes imbalance and strain.*

r. *Keep your weight back, hold the item close and lengthen upwards.*

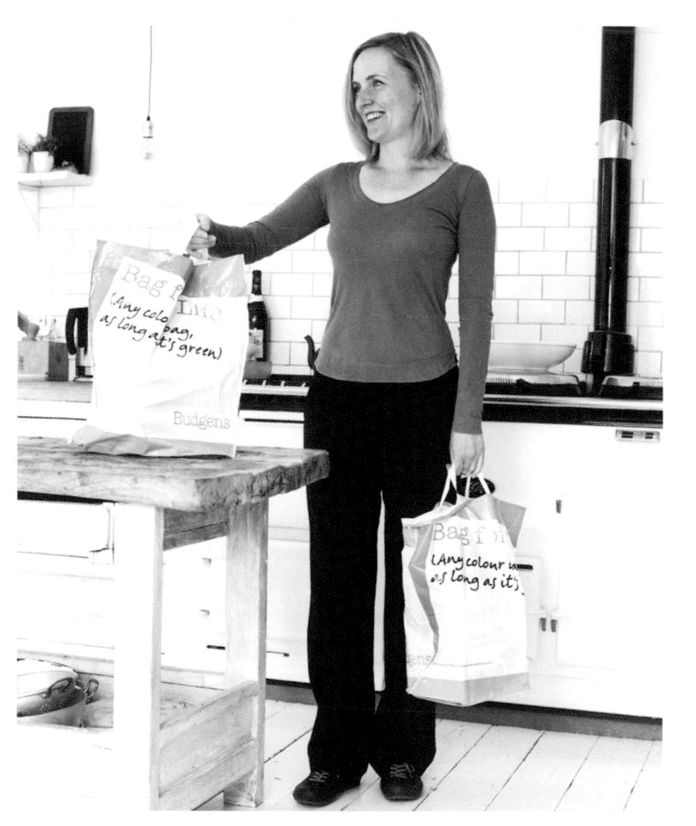

Carry two lighter bags rather than one heavy bag.

HELPFUL TIPS

- Carry as little as possible. Leave things out of the bag if they are not needed today.
- Wear a back pack or shoulder bag worn diagonally across your spine to spread the weight.
- Avoid leaning forward. 'Direct' your neck to be free and your head to go upward.
- If carrying a heavy box in front of you, come back on your ankles to compensate.
- Carry the load as close to your body as possible.
- Carry two smaller bags, one in each hand, rather than one large bag. Spread the load.
- Keep your neck free and breathe.
- Get someone else to carry it!

Lunge

We can use the lunge as a 'position of mechanical advantage' that can encourage an enhancement of our 'use' and co-ordination. It is most commonly seen in a thrusting attack in swordsmanship but it can also be helpful in vacuum cleaning, pushing a pram, mowing the lawn or sawing a piece of wood. You can see children playing using lunge and 'Monkey' positions. It is a means of moving your weight forward and retreating efficiently and deftly. In essence, it enables movement with the least amount of strain on the body, protecting the working parts and avoiding pain while enabling us to make the most of ourselves in activities. It is worth practising the following exercises.

Exercise – Lunge

Note: This procedure is best done under the supervision of a qualified Alexander Technique teacher.

We will do this exercise in several separate small stages. Pause and 'inhibit' between each movement to think 'how' you are doing it. Use a 'means-whereby' approach to your movements. Think first.

›› Stand with your feet together and free your neck. Bring your weight back over your ankles so you are not leaning. 'Direct' your head forward and upward and your back to lengthen and widen.

›› Turn your right foot outward by about 45 degrees and place its heel into the instep of your left foot so it is slightly in front and at an angle.

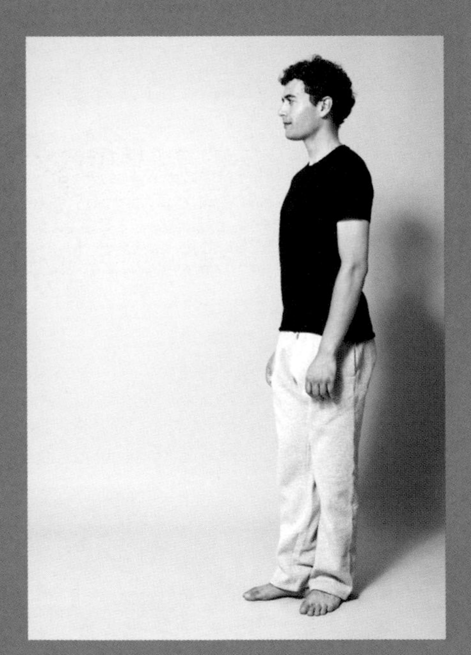

Place right heel into the instep of the left foot. Turn bodily to the right.

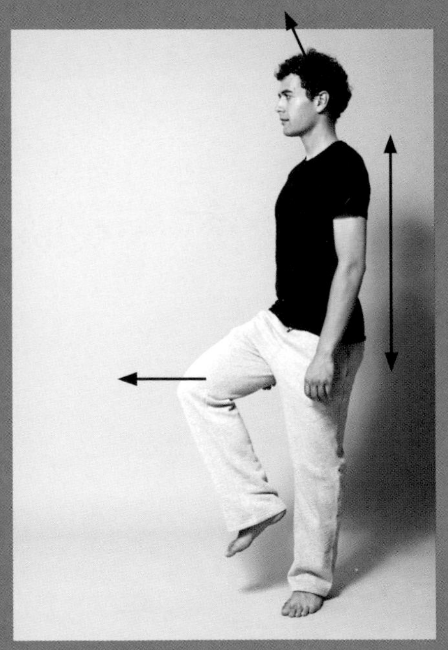

Direct upwards and send your right knee forwards.

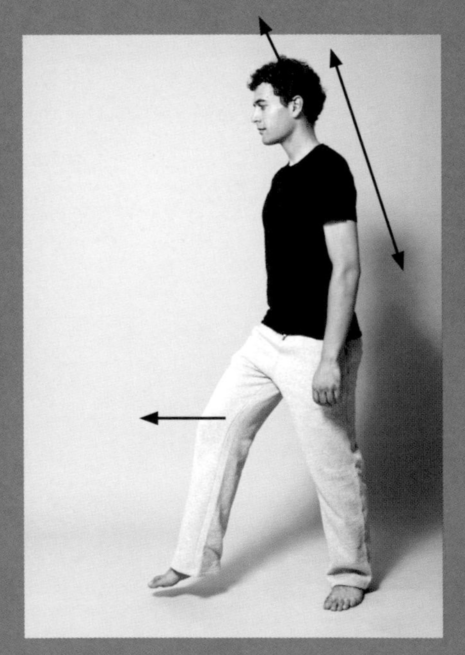

Free your neck and lengthen as you move.

- Turn your whole upper body to face right in the direction of your angled foot. Your body, neck and head should turn 'in one piece'. Do not disturb the head/neck/back relationship.

- Bring your body weight back over the heel of your left foot so there is less weight on your right foot. Pay particular attention to allowing your lower and upper back to be back over your left ankle.

- In a moment you will move your right foot forward by 45cm (18in) in line with your foot, but you will do so by doing two key things: you will 'direct' your head forward and upward to lengthen from your left heel, while at the same time lift your right knee and send it forward in the same line as your foot. 'Inhibit' moving instantly to think how you are doing it. Your right foot will come off the floor and land 45cm (18in) in front and to the side of your left foot. You will bodily face the direction of movement and arrive in a new position leaning forward over your right foot. Your left foot remains where it is.

Note:
Your head and knee must lead the movement.
Do not push your hips forward. There should be a straight line from your occipital joint of your neck down through your hip to your left ankle. This remains constant during the whole movement.
Avoid your head pulling backward as you move. Think free and forward and up.
Your left leg should remain straight at all times. Keep your left heel on the floor so you feel a nice stretch up the back of your leg.
Now you extend the exercise by moving your body weight from one foot to another. Leave your feet where they are and bring your whole body 'in one piece' back over your left foot so your right leg straightens and your left knee bends. Your body should become vertical in this position. Now transfer your weight forward again over your right heel, your body will lean at an angle.
Your head/neck/back relationship should not alter with this movement. Keep your neck free and your head 'going' upward. Avoid hollowing your back.

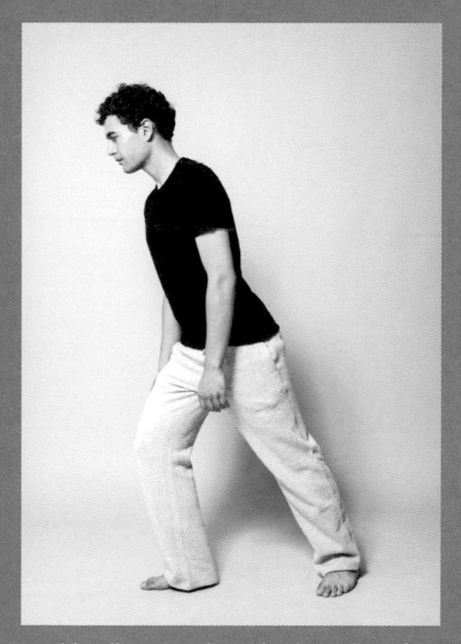

Avoid pulling your head backwards. Left heel remains on the floor.

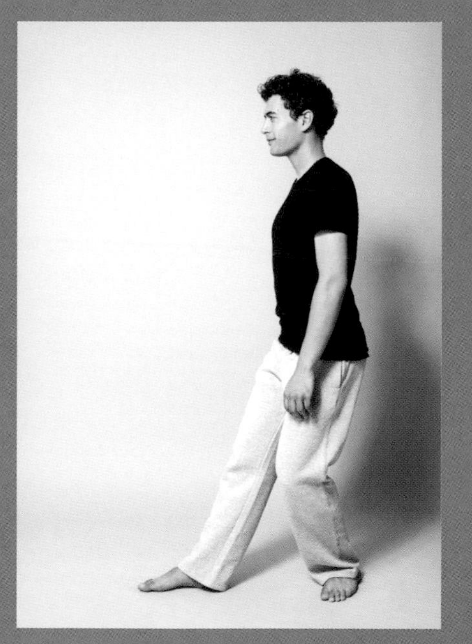

Straighten your right leg and bend your left. Your body should become vertical.

The lunge can be done in the opposite direction. To do so, follow the above guidelines but move your left foot forward and away 45 degrees from your right foot and turn bodily to the left

NB: The lunge can be performed in two main ways. The photo sequence shows an exaggerated movement, so that the principle can be clearly seen. In normal life, the lunge is performed as a simple glide so the foot moving forward does not come so far off the floor.

Crawling

Another very helpful process is to do some crawling on all fours as it uses your muscles differently and can improve their co-ordination. This procedure is helpful for all people, particularly if you suffer from back pain and during pregnancy. It is also a great exercise for tight wrists and hands as it opens them out. You will need a good length of carpeted floor. The exercise should only be performed for a few minutes before returning to standing.

Exercise – Crawling

Note: This is best done under the supervision of an Alexander Technique teacher.

Part A – Getting down into crawling position

- Stand evenly on both feet and free your neck. 'Inhibit' getting down on your knees until you have centred yourself and brought your weight back over your ankles.
- Put one hand on the back of a chair to steady yourself.
- Put your right foot behind you and lower yourself down onto your right knee.
- Bring your left knee down so they are spaced under your hips.
- Kneel tall then allow your hips to come backward and fold forward keeping a tall back so you land on your hands in front of you.
- Place the palms of your hands under your shoulders so they are spaced out and fingers pointing forward.
- Your hands should be sufficiently spaced from your knees so your arms and thighs are vertical. Do not increase or decrease this distance. You should be rather like a table.
- Look at the floor so your head is not pulled backward.
- 'Direct' the crown of your head forward toward a far-away wall and 'direct' your sacrum (the base of the spine) backward so your back lengthens.
- Avoid hollowing your back; this should remain as flat as possible.

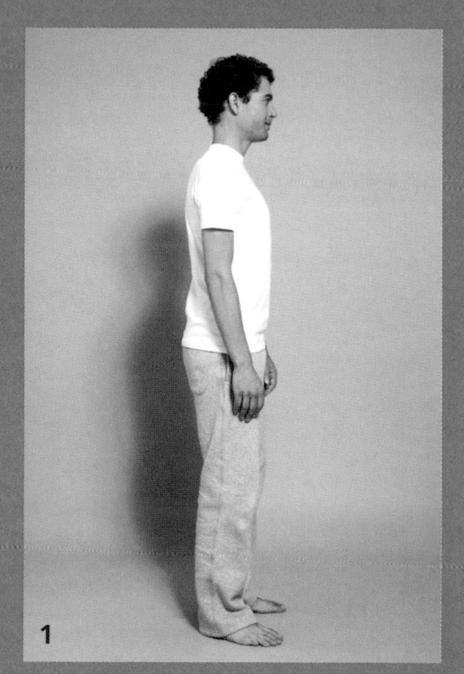

Inhibit rushing to give time to free your neck and direct upwards.

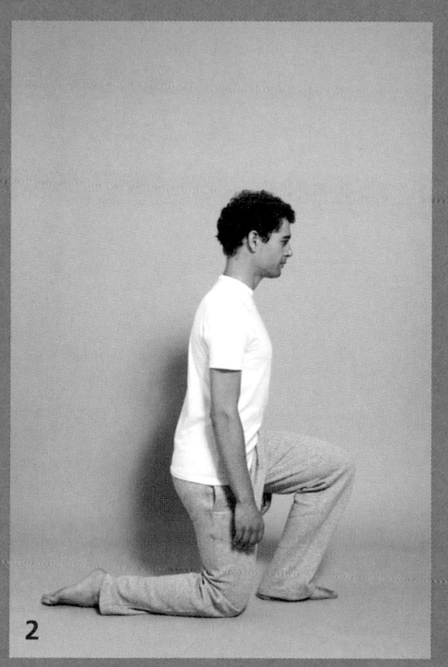

Put your right foot behind and lower yourself onto your right knee.

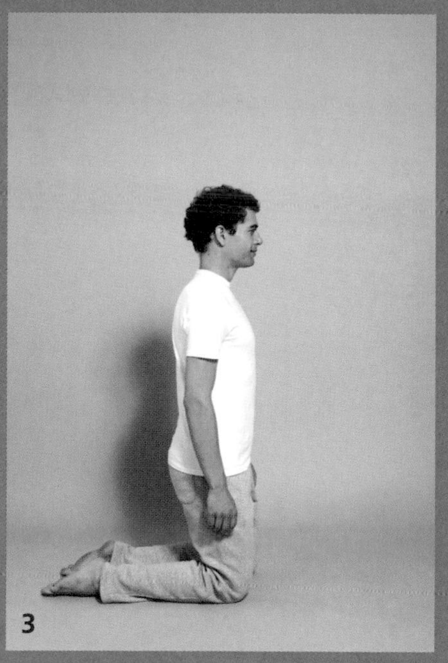

Kneel tall, free your neck and direct upward.

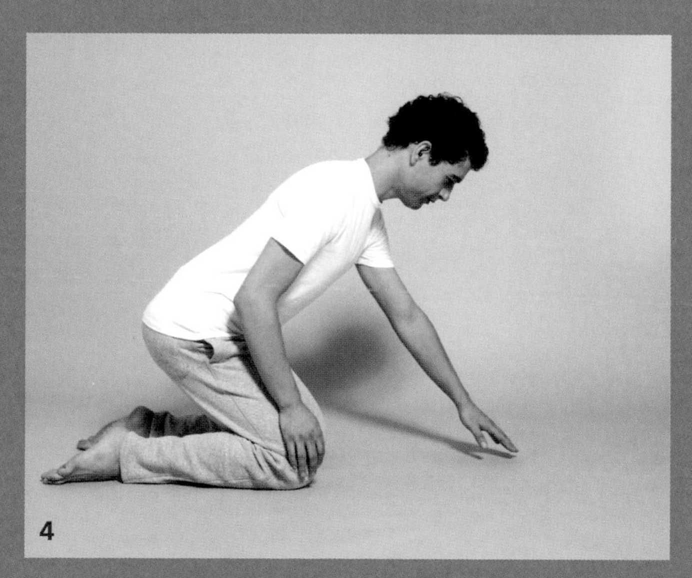

Allow your hips to come backwards and place your hands in front of you.

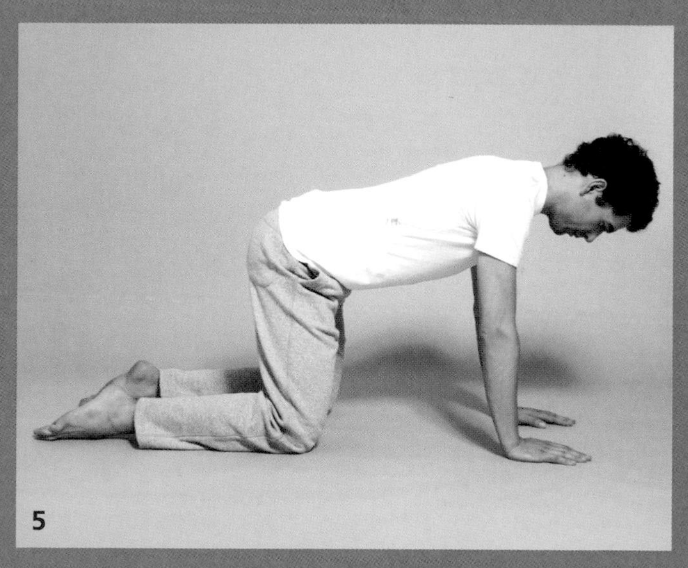

Position hands under shoulders, knees under hips.

Avoid Problems

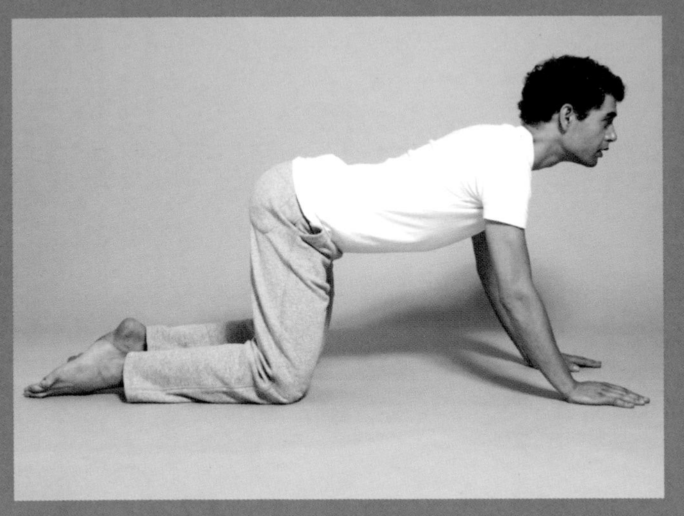

Do not hollow your back or pull your head backwards.

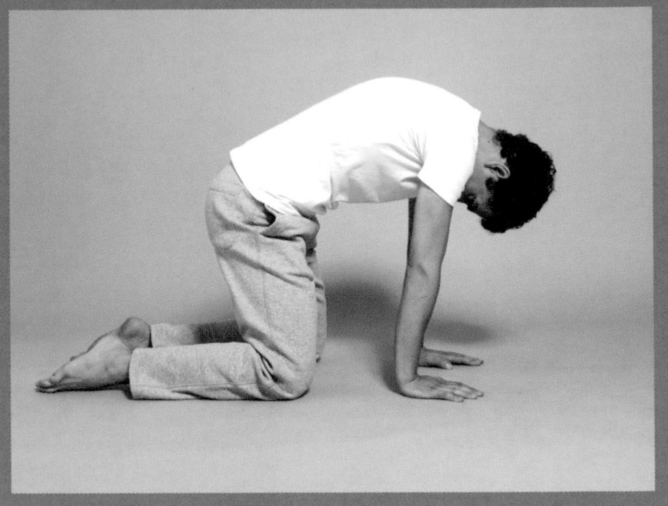

Do not place your hands too close to your knees or round your back.

Exercise – Rock backward and forward slowly

›› Now you can rock gently backward and forward very slowly. First lead with your head to lengthen in your back as you move forward. Then you lead with your sacrum, to lengthen your back as you come backward. Think of lengthening from the tailbone to the crown of your head. Enjoy the movement and sense of length. Become familiar with rocking slowly in this way before proceeding to crawling. Remember to look at the floor.

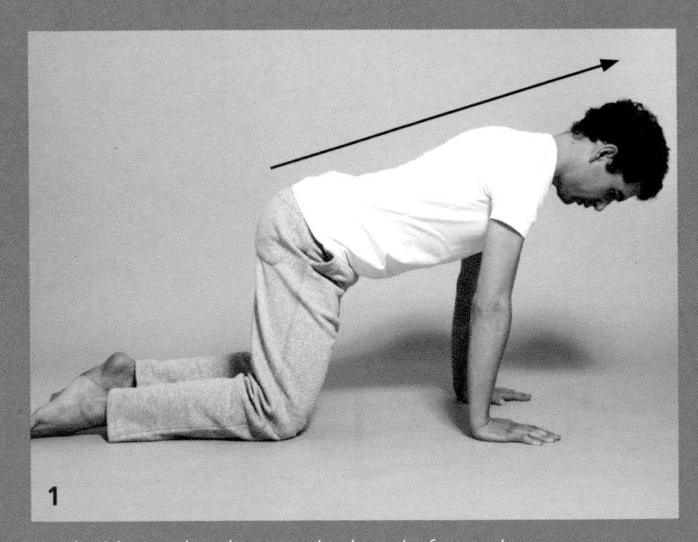

Lead with your head so your body rocks forward.

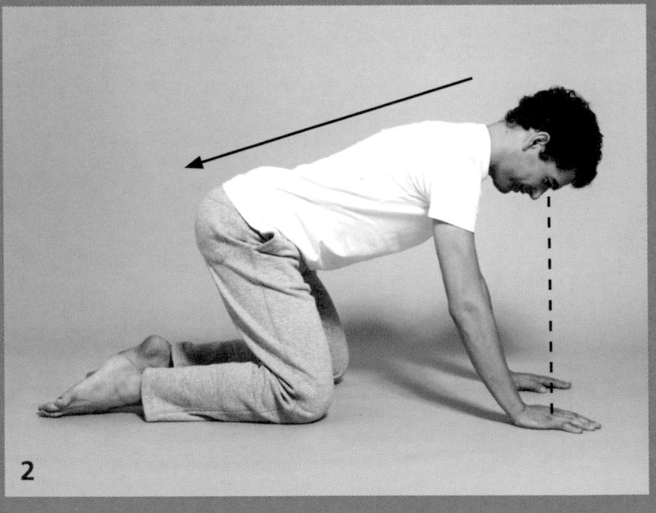

Lead with your bottom so your body rocks backward.

Part B – Crawling in four-time (Homolateral movement – asymmetrical movement of one arm and leg on the same side)

- Establish a stable and lengthening pose on hands and knees and rock slowly backward and forward as described opposite. Remember to look at the floor.
- To crawl, lead with your head so you sway forward and at the same time slide your left knee 10cm (4in) forward in a straight line.
- Pause and then lead with your head so you place your left hand 10cm (4in) forward.
- Pause to think, lead with your head and slide your right knee forward 20cm (8in) so it passes your left knee.
- Pause to think, lead with your head and move your right hand forward 20cm (8in) so it passes your left hand.
- Now you move your left knee again 20cm (8in).
- Then your left hand 20cm (8in).
- Right knee 20cm (8in).
- Right hand 20cm (8in).

Establish an even rhythm of movement 'knee, hand, knee, hand' similar to the rhythm of a ticking clock. Small steps are better than long ones.

Return to standing (this is the same process as getting up from Semi-supine Position (see page 100).

(Continued on next page)

Tips

›› Always look at the floor and lead with the crown of your head.
›› Don't let your knees catch up with your hands as this will round your back.
›› Keep your knees apart under your hips and slide them forward in a straight line, neither inward nor outward.
›› Keep your back long and flat.
›› Look at each hand as you move it by first looking with your eyes then gently turning your head left and right.
›› Breathe.

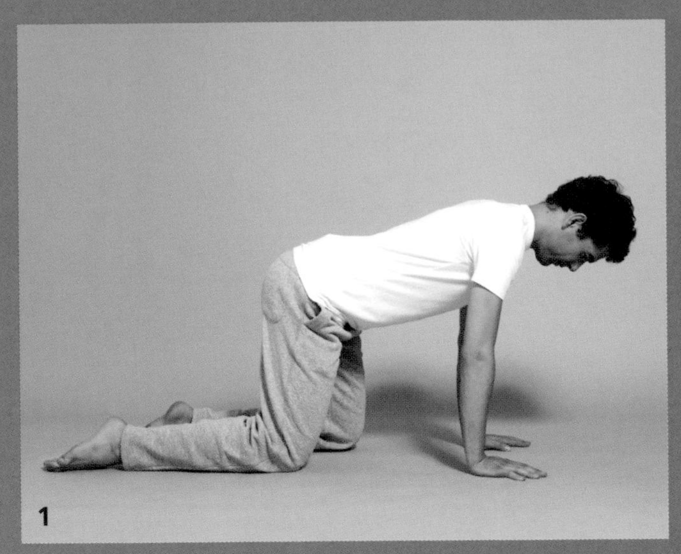

1

Move hand and knee independently. Send your head forward to lengthen. Slide your left knee 10cm (4in) forward.

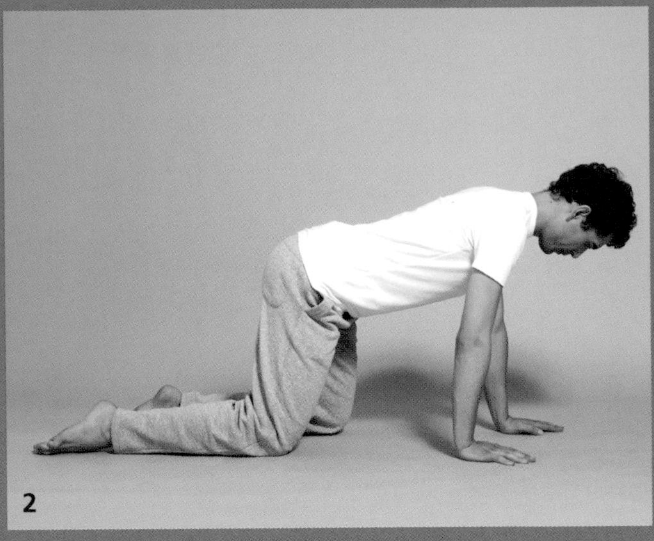

2

Send your head forward. Move your left hand forward by 10cm (4in).

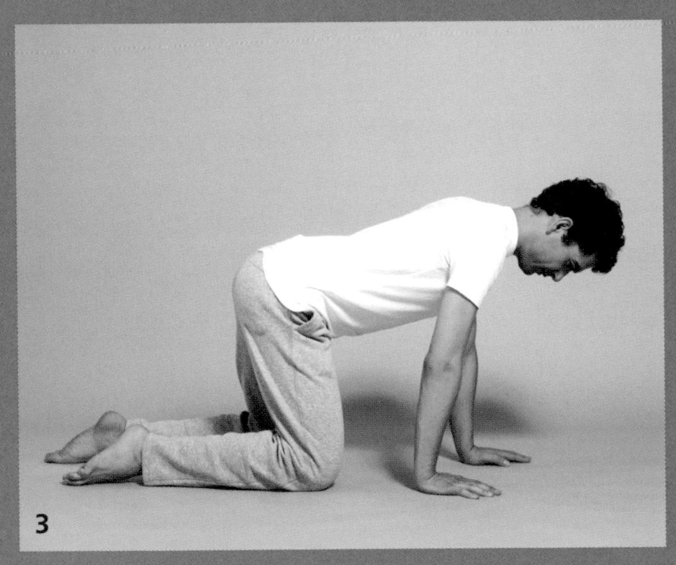

3

Send your head forward. Slide your right knee forward 20cm (8in).

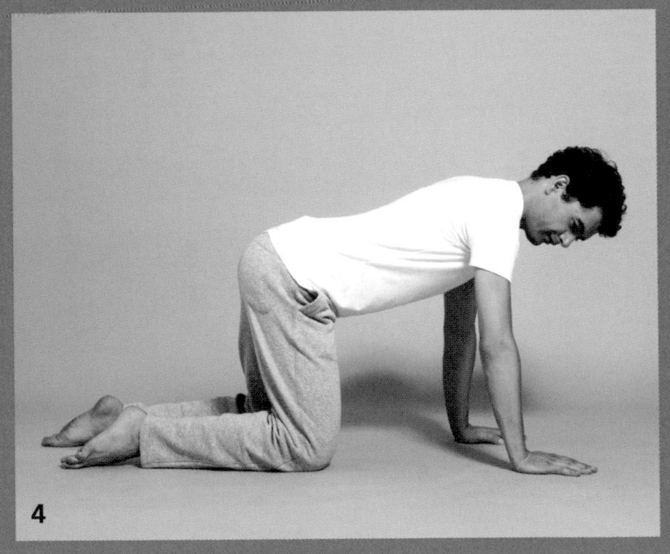

4

Lead with your head. Place your right hand forward 20cm (8in).

Crawling in four-time as described above happens when we crawl slowly, but as soon as we increase speed, the natural inclination will be to change to cross pattern, two-time crawling.

Exercise – Crawling in two-time (Cross pattern – simultaneous movement of hand and knee diagonally opposite one another)

- Establish a good crawling position as described above. Take your time.
- Lead with your head as you slide your left knee and lift your right hand simultaneously forward by 10cm (4in)
- Lead with your head as you slide your right knee and lift your left hand simultaneously forward by 20cm (8in) so they pass the left knee and right hand.
- Lead with your head as you slide your left knee and lift your right hand forward.
- Continue, leading with your head. Establish an even rhythm.
- Return to standing as previously described.

After returning to standing, pause and bring your weight back over your ankles. Free your neck and 'direct' yourself to lengthen and widen. Allow your weight to go down through your heels so you feel grounded.

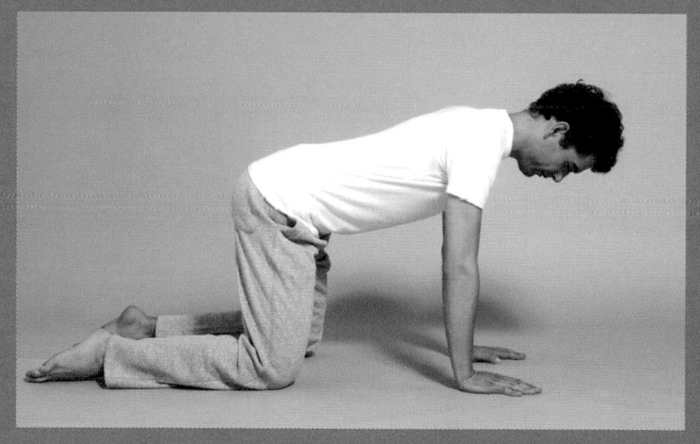

Start with hands under shoulders, knees under hips.

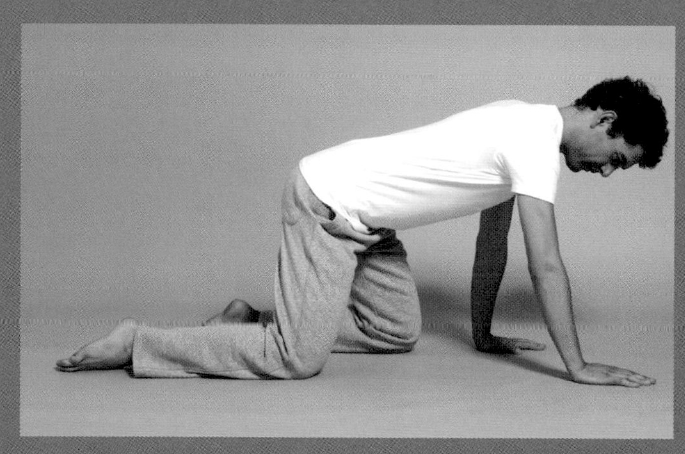

Send your head forwards. Move left knee and right hand simultaneously.

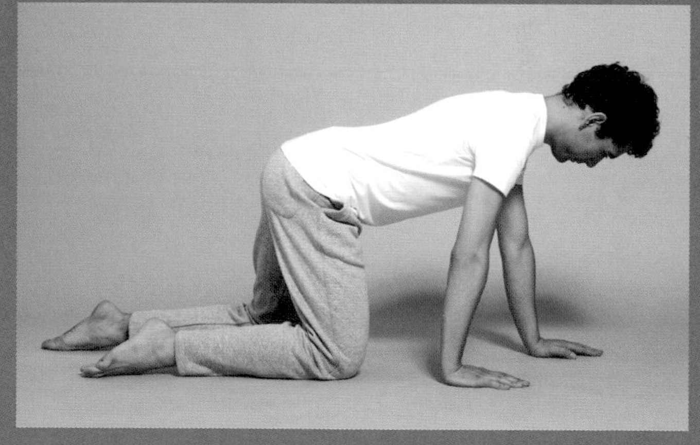

Lead with your head. Move right knee and left hand simultaneously.

Running

Running is a wonderful way of keeping fit and healthy but can be problematic if we run in such a way as to increase strain on our back, neck and legs. If we experience back pain when running, it is because our running style is inefficient and we are probably off balance and using excessive effort. To help our running be a joy rather than a pain, we should run lightly; if we can hear our feet pounding on the path, we will probably cause joint and back problems in the future.

The principles of the Alexander Technique apply to running as well as any other activity, and can help us achieve more speed with less effort while also avoiding injury.

The key thing is that you should lengthen in stature as you run; your head should be directed forward and upward, your back lengthened and widened. Your knees should also lead each stride, not your feet. We should also ensure we do not shorten in our front, which can be a tendency when we tire, causing us to plod rather heavily. We should not 'come down' as we run, but 'go up'.

Experiment by running with shorter strides. This technique will help avoid a braking action that occurs if your stride is long. It is better to take more short strides and do so freely than fewer long strides.

HELPFUL TIPS

Use a 'means-whereby' approach to running. Don't 'end-gain'. Think.

›› Before running, pause. 'Inhibit' launching forward to give yourself time to free your neck and 'direct' your head forward and upward.

›› Moving into a run is similar to the lunge. If you are going to stride forward with your right leg, you should 'direct' your head forward and up away from your left heel to make the stride.

›› Point each knee forward as you stride. The knees should lead, not the feet.

›› Look ahead without pulling your head backward. If you pull your head back, you are more likely to hollow your back.

›› Do not lean too far forward as you run. Keep your weight back a bit and think your head upward.

›› Forearms should be horizontal and move forward and backward opposite to each stride. Do not move your arms across your body, but parallel to the direction you are running in, like railway tracks.

›› Keep your wrists straight, hands gently curled so your arm movement is led by your knuckles.

›› When you run slowly, your heel will touch the ground first, if you run at moderate pace your mid-foot touches first and only if you are sprinting will each foot land on the toes.

›› Try to run quietly by giving your directions.

›› Stop regularly to re-establish your poise and free your neck. 'Inhibit' carrying on with stubbornness.

›› If you are tiring 'stop'. There is nothing more likely to cause back trouble than running when you are over-tired.

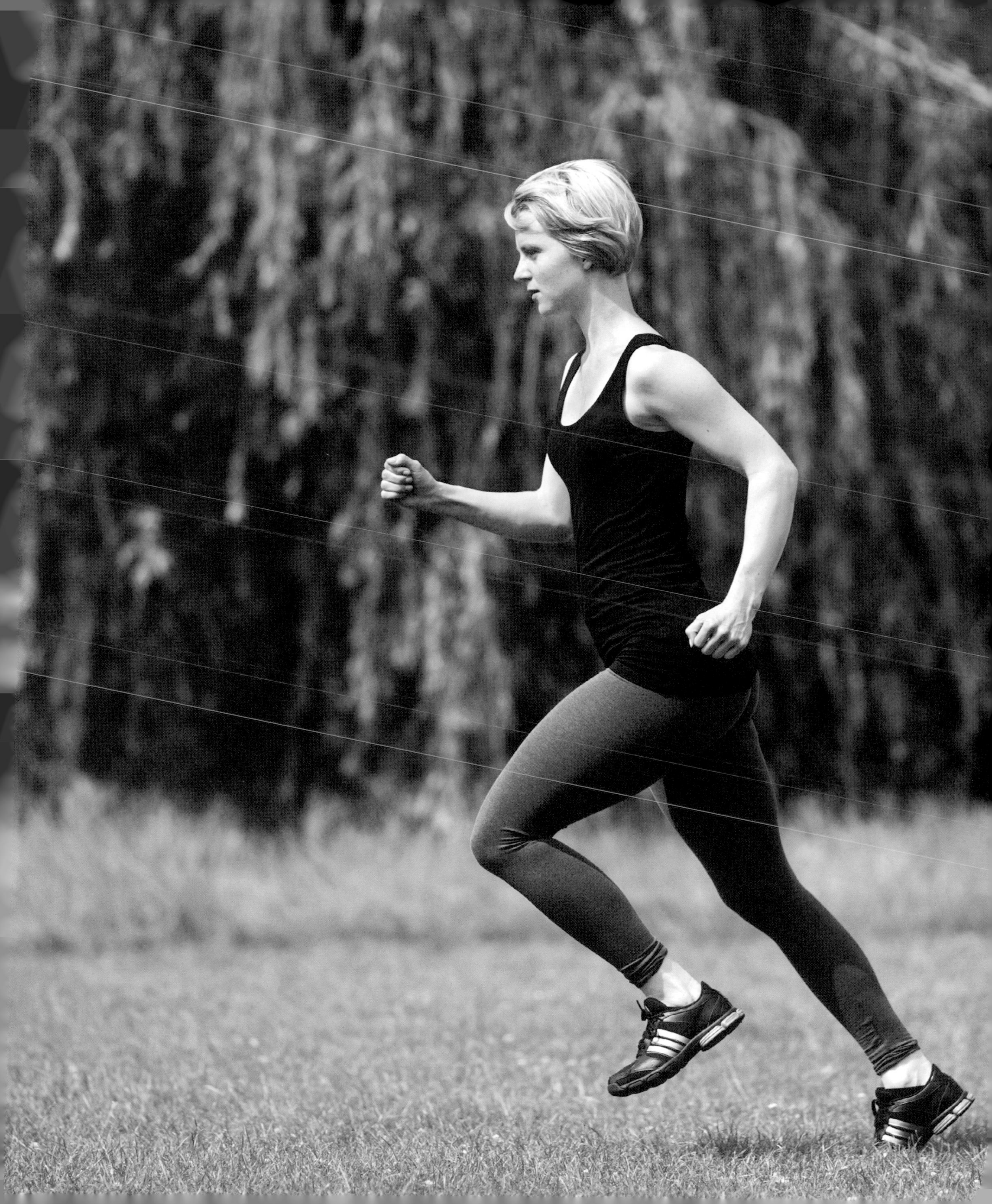

Pregnancy

The Alexander Technique can be extremely useful throughout pregnancy in helping you cope with the rapid changes occurring to your body in a healthy and pain-free way.

Having Alexander lessons before pregnancy will help avoid problems but it is helpful at any stage of pregnancy as it can be an important contribution to a comfortable, natural birth.

One of the most common tendencies during pregnancy is to allow the growing weight of the baby to pull your hips forward and arch your back. This causes compression of the hips and lumbar spine and a downward dragging of your entire body. In later months this tendency can become more exaggerated and cause severe backache. The worst thing you can do when experiencing back pain is put your hands on your lower back and arch your back further, which

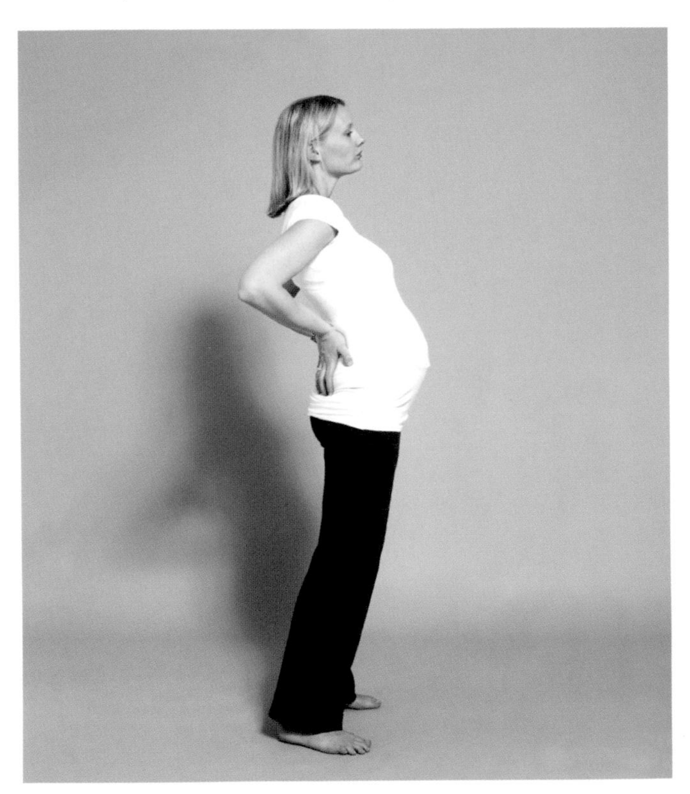

Exercise – Standing

- Stand with your feet spaced apart under your hips.
- Bring your hips back so they are not pushed forward. A straight line should be drawn from the ankles through the hips to the occipital joint in your neck.
- Let your head roll forward on top of your spine to free your neck. 'Direct' your back to lengthen.
- 'Direct' lower back to widen and open out.
- Allow your whole body weight to adjust to the baby in front by coming back from your ankles without changing the alignment.

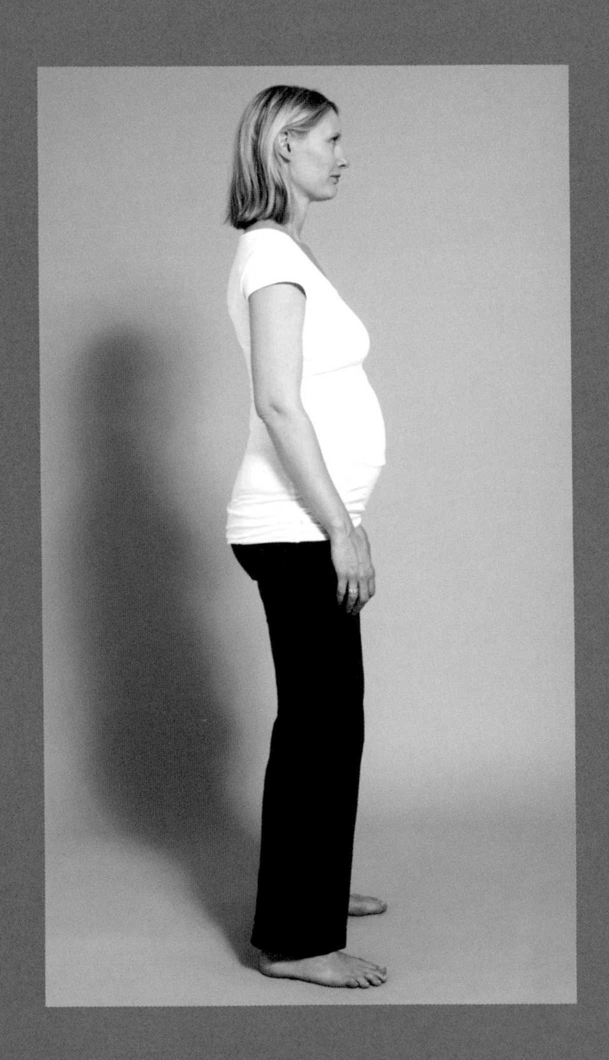

puts your whole body out of natural alignment and balance. The key is to help your body maintain its natural alignment by conscious awareness. When suffering from pain, you might react in a 'startle pattern' reflex by stiffening your neck, pulling your head back off balance and shortening your front. Try to inhibit these tendencies by consciously releasing your neck by letting your head roll forward, let go of the tension in your shoulders, 'direct' your head forward and upward, release your jaw and tongue and keep breathing.

When standing, you should ideally allow your body weight to come back from your ankles without arching your back (see exercise 'Adapting your balance to cope with carrying a weight' on page 136).

Lying down on the floor in Semi-supine Position (page 98) can be very helpful for relieving lower back pain, however this procedure may not be comfortable later in pregnancy as your baby and uterus exert pressure on the large blood vessels in the lumbar back. A way of relieving this discomfort may be to put your legs onto a chair when doing the procedure.

Monkey Position (page 108) is one of the most helpful and dynamic postures you can adopt to relieve your back pain. In later months this position can provide more internal space for your baby and encourage the head to enter the pelvic opening, adopting the optimal position ready for birth.

Crawling, as described on page 142, is a most helpful way of relieving back pain during pregnancy as it takes the weight of the baby off your lower spine. In later months crawling as an exercise can encourage your baby to move into an anterior position and is great preparation both physically and mentally for the process of childbirth.

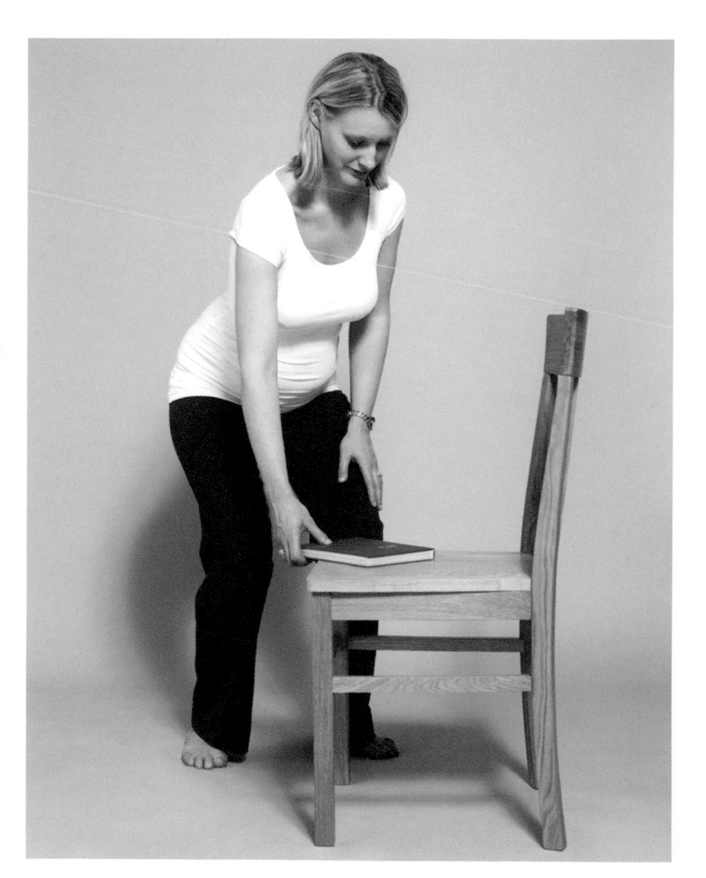

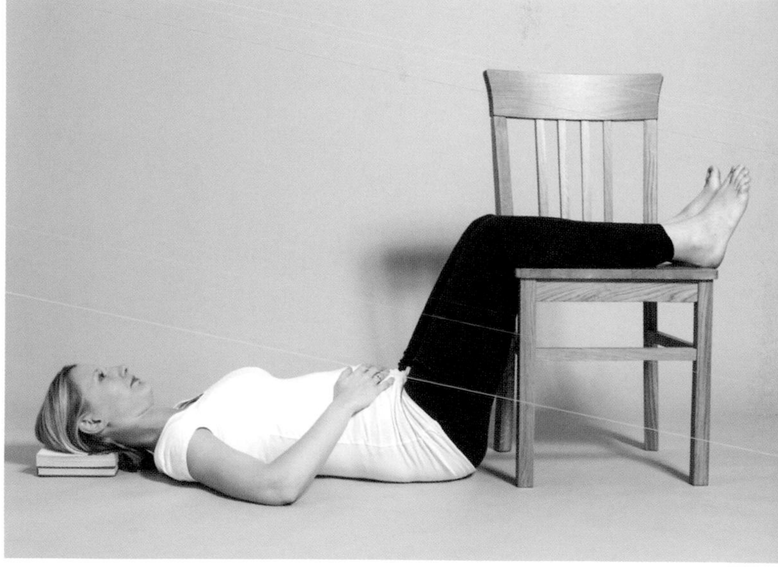

l. *Monkey position (page 108) with feet well spaced.*

r. *Semi-supine position (page 98) with lower legs on a chair to relieve pressure on back.*

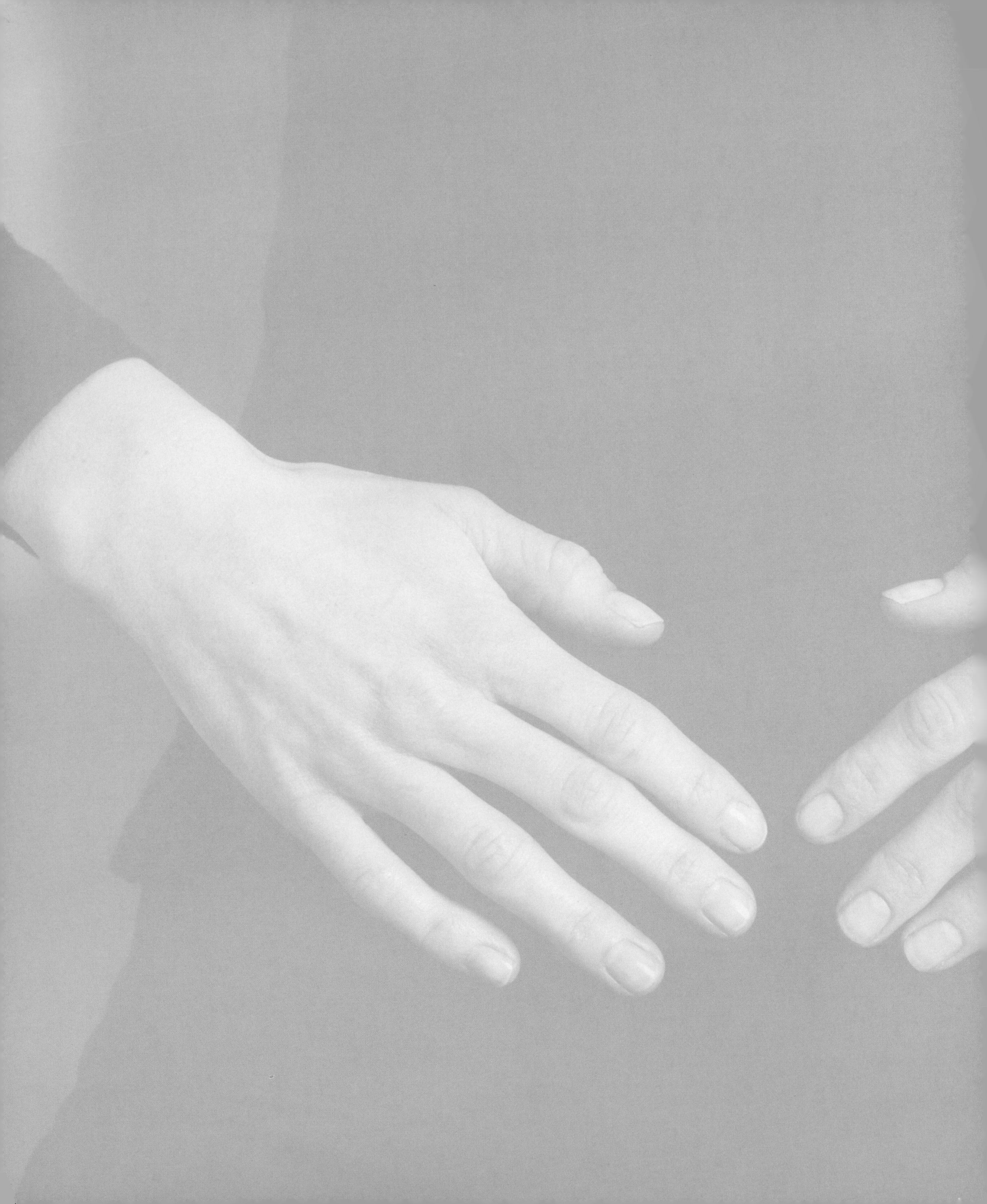

BREATHING

6

Breathing

Many experts believe that a lack of oxygen in human cell tissue is linked to a range of health problems and diseases. Therefore it's clearly important that we do not allow our habits to interfere with this vital process. Oxygen feeds our muscle tissues in poise and activity and is a major part of collagen, which gives our skin, ligaments and tendons their elasticity. Collagen accounts for 30 per cent of body protein and is made up of oxygen, nitrogen and hydrogen. Water is made of oxygen and hydrogen and the hydrogen helps to bind our atoms together. As we are composed of approximately 70 per cent water, it's clearly important that we drink sufficient quantities on a daily basis to help maintain the elasticity of our soft tissue.

Any form of unnecessary tension tends to interfere with breathing; you may notice that you hold your breath in certain stressful situations as posture habits often reduce the regularity of our breathing. We may still be alive but if we breathed more regularly and efficiently we could be even more alive! Breathing involves both the movement of the diaphragm and the ribs. The intercostal muscles around our ribs can become tight with postural habits preventing easy movement. This also affects the movement of our diaphragm which connects to the anterior side of our lumbar spine causing it to become stuck. Freeing up this area improves blood supply and movement both of which are conducive to the healthy functioning of your back.

Breathing is not a separate function of our body, but is linked inextricably to our whole posture. F.M. Alexander discovered that habitual tension interfered with his breathing. He evolved what we now know as the Alexander Technique as a means of overcoming his vocal and breathing problems, and even became known as the 'Breathing Man' in Sydney and Melbourne in the late nineteenth century.

If left without interference breathing will work perfectly well of its own accord. It is a vital life function automatically controlled by the autonomic nervous system. Our brain monitors levels of oxygen, hydrogen, nitrogen, carbon dioxide and other gases to ensure adequate and not excessive amounts of each are present in the body for it to function well in different circumstances and activities. We should not try and 'control' our breathing, rather we need to leave it alone for it to function of its own accord. All the guidelines in this book will help free up your breathing. Breathing is an extensive topic and requires much more space than is available in this book, however I want to suggest one procedure that will likely benefit not only your back but also your overall health.

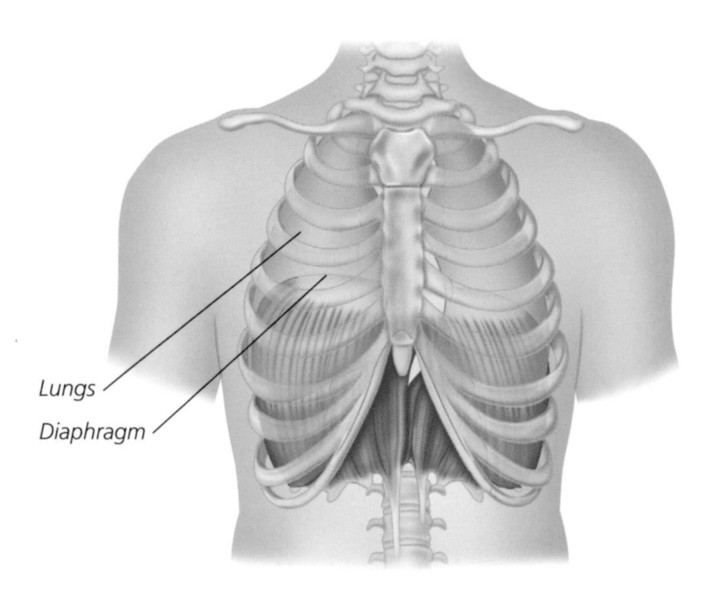

The lungs are located in our back and are moved by the ribs and diaphragm.

Exercise - The Whispered Ahh

This procedure is deceptively simple. It can be performed sitting, but preferably standing, with maximum attention to ensure you gain the potential benefits.

- First 'inhibit'. Bring yourself up to your full stature by freeing your neck, 'direct' your head forward and upward and think of lengthening and widening.
- Allow your head to balance freely on top of your spine. With your lips closed, let your jaw be free by allowing it to hang loosely with a small space between the back molar teeth. Let your jaw be 'slung' freely.
- Place the tip of your tongue behind your lower teeth and let it lie relaxed on the floor of your mouth.
- In a moment you are going to make the sound 'Ahh' in a gentle whisper, under your breath. The process of making this sound is rather like breathing hot air onto a mirror to remove a mark. It is a whispered sound, not vocalised at all. A good description of the sound is what you would hear if you put a seashell to your ear to hear the ocean.
- Think of something to smile about.
- Allow your jaw to fall open a little and, with the smile, make a breathy sound 'Ahh' that lasts around 4 seconds.
- Close your mouth and allow the air to return to your lungs through your nose without sniffing.
- Perform the Whispered Ahh again, making the sound as smooth and clear as you can. Use the minimum of effort. The sound should be quiet and gentle, without force.
- Perform the procedure 6–8 times but no more. If you feel slightly dizzy, stop immediately.
- Remember, this is not a method of breathing, but a procedure to be performed just a few times to stimulate the healthy movement of your ribs and diaphragm.

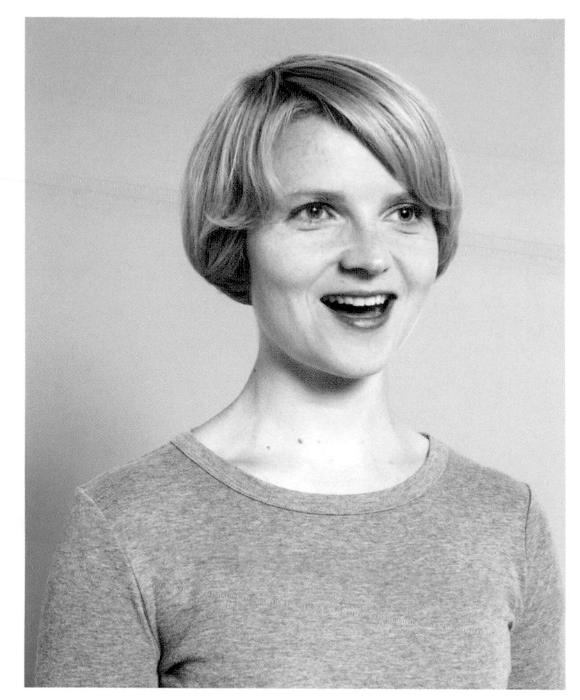

The Whispered Ahh.

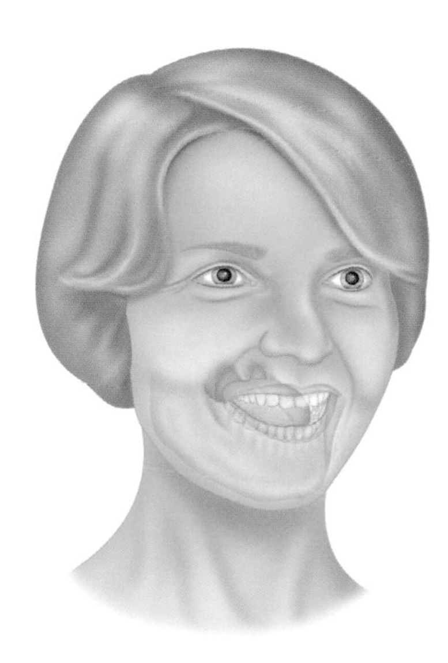

Let the tip of your tongue lie behind your lower teeth.

Remember that breathing is a natural process; don't try and breathe – just let it happen. If you notice during the day that you are holding your breath, breathe out first as this stimulates your *natural breathing*.

Conclusion

The Alexander Technique can be truly transformational. How much it can transform your life is dependent on the degree to which you can inhibit the tendencies to 'do'. As the majority of our problems relating to posture and backache are the result of 'doing the wrong thing' and losing our natural co-ordination, the ceasing of these habits is fundamental to change. It is easy to fall into the pattern of doing something to rectify a problem: we try harder, we change how we're 'holding' ourselves, we pull ourselves up straight, we push our shoulders back. But with this rather crude approach all we succeed in doing is simply superimposing further negative behaviours on top of those that already exist, and the problems become even more complex and ingrained. It is all this 'doing' that gets in the way of a system that is far more subtle and sophisticated than we can ever hope to fully understand. Learning to 'stop', to give ourselves time and to 'inhibit' our negative patterns is key to bringing about the change we want.

Postural problems are due mostly to poor co-ordination. Our muscles are no longer as finely tuned as they once were, some are over-tense and others are under-performing, and this is evident in the simple observation of our out-of-balance poise in the mirror. F.M. Alexander pointed out quite rightly that, 'The right thing will do itself', but we need to let it. This means 'getting out of the way of ourselves' and ceasing all the 'wrong doing'. It involves 'inhibiting' so we gain release from unwanted tensions and patterns, not the habit-controlled contractions that come from simply trying to 'do it correctly'. What we really want is the sensation of release, and that cannot be 'done'; it needs to be allowed.

Only when we stop our misguided efforts and put ourselves into a more neutral state can we then give mental instructions via the Alexander Technique 'directions' that will bring about a new and better co-ordination. It is the thinking that counts, not the effort. The giving of correct 'directions' communicated by our thinking can transform our co-ordination and the function of our whole mechanism. Through our thinking, by Inhibition and Direction, we can bring about a release from habit and experience the joy of freely expanding in stature. The sensation can be unusual, uplifting and somewhat vaguely familiar. This is because we are reviving the natural poise we enjoyed as young children; the difference is that we are now achieving it consciously. It is re-learning.

You can change your co-ordination, your poise and even your outlook in life by simply stopping the wrong thing and by thinking. Backache can then become a thing of the past and will never return for reasons of poor posture as long as you continue using the principles of the Alexander Technique. Take some Alexander lessons and follow the guidelines in this book on a daily basis and you will never look back.

References and Further Reading

[1] Palmer KT, Walsh K, et al. Back pain in Britain: comparison of two prevalence surveys at an interval of 10 years BMJ 2000;320:1577-1578.

[2] Alexander, F. M., *Man's Supreme Intelligence*, 1910.

[3] http://www.painclinic.org/aboutpain-painmechanisms.htm

[4] http://www.painclinic.org/aboutpain-painmechanisms.htm

[5] Alexander, F. M., *The Use of the Self*, 1932

by F. M. Alexander:
Man's Supreme Inheritance
Constructive Conscious Control of the Individual
The Use of the Self
The Universal Constant in Living
Articles and Lectures
Aphorisms

Freedom to Change, Frank Pierce Jones
Collected Writings on the Alexander Technique, Frank Pierce Jones
Thinking Aloud, Walter Carrington
The Act of Living, Walter Carrington
Personally Speaking, Walter Carrington and Sean Carey
Explaining the Alexander Technique, Walter Carrington and Sean Carey
F. Matthias Alexander – The Man and His Work, Lulie Westfeldt
The Alexander Technique Birth Book, I. Machover and A. & J. Drake
F. M. - The Life of Frederick Matthias Alexander, Michael Bloch
Up From Down Under, Rosslyn McLeod
Curiosity Recaptured, Jerry Sontag
Voice and the Alexander Technique, Jane Heirich
Skill and Poise, Raymond A. Dart
The Art of Swimming, Steven Shaw & Armand D'Angour (for more information on the Shaw Method of Swimming visit www.swimshawmethod.com)
Body Learning, Michael Gelb
Indirect Procedures (A musician's guide to the Alexander Technique), Pedro de Alcantara
Atlas of the Skeletal Muscles, Robert J. Stone & Judith A. Stone.
The Complete Illustrated Guide to Alexander Technique, Glynn MacDonald
The Alexander Technique Manual, Richard Brennan
Body, Breath & Being, Carolyn Nicholls
Illustrated Physiology, McNaught and Callander
Mind and Muscle, Elizabeth Langford

By the same author
Perfect Poise, Perfect Life, Noël Kingsley

The full 2008 *BMJ* study can be found by following the link entitled 'Back Pain Study' at www.stat.org.uk.

Useful Contacts

To find a qualified Alexander Technique teacher local to your area in the UK please visit www.stat.org.uk or call 0207 482 5135. For teacher in countries other than the UK, visit www.stat.or.uk and links will be found for Affiliated Societies Overseas.

Index

Acknowledgements

I wish to pay tribute to F.M. Alexander, the originator of the Alexander Technique, the method I feel so lucky and privileged to have been able to use all my adult life having been introduced to it in 1972.

I also wish to convey a special thanks to the late Walter Carrington, a protégé and assistant of Alexander himself for twenty years and his wife Dilys Carrington, both founding directors of the Constructive Teaching Centre, London, where I trained as a teacher of the Alexander Technique and whose training exercises or 'games' as they are known have been incorporated into this book. I also wish to thank them for their enormous kindness and generosity. Thank you to all the other Alexander teachers and students I have worked with for sharing their knowledge, expertise and skill. Thank you to the late Jeanne Day and her husband Aksel Haahr who gave me my first Alexander lessons, also to Marjory Barlow and Peggy Williams. Thank you to Gerald Foley for his critical advice, Vivien Mackie and Charlotte Rolleston-Smith. I would also like to acknowledge the thousands of people with whom I have had the pleasure and experience of working.

A special thank you goes to my partner Miranda for her love, her unceasing and tireless support and encouragement and for just being great.

Thank you to Eddie Jacobs for his wonderful photography, Louise Leffler for her superb design work and Amanda Williams for her lovely illustrations. Also thank you to the Alexander teachers who kindly agreed to model for us: David López Veneros, Elisabeth Dahl, Susanna Scouller and Angus Antley, and also to Angus's son Jones, Michelle Rowley and her son Marlie, Peter French and Gemma John. Many thanks to my wonderful agent Sheila Ableman for her tremendous experience and advice. Thank you also to Judith Hannam and the team at Kyle Cathie Ltd, and in particular Catharine Robertson for her superb handling and management of the project.

Last but not least, a special thank you to my Dad for his love, his unceasing enthusiastic encouragement and his inspiration. I am immeasurably grateful to Dad and my late mother for introducing me to the Alexander Technique when I was a young man.

Photo credits

p.12 CHASSENET CHASSENET/BSIP Medical
p.20 (l) Andy Crawford; (r) Ronald Wittek/Picture Press
p.21 MBI/Alamy
p.22 (t) Stockbyte; (b) John Van Decker/Alamy
p.23 (l) Tim Graham/Alamy; (r) Alamy Premium/Alamy
p.28 & 29 (all) The Society of Teachers of the Alexander Technique, London
p.30 (l–r) Jamie Grill Photography; Andersen Ross; Jamie Grill Photography; George Doyle
p.31 Getty Images
p.32 (t) Image Source/Alamy; (b) Andre Gravel
p.33 PBNJ Productions
p.34 Ojo Images
p.38 Sunset Boulevard/Corbis
p.39 (l) Photoalto; (r) Image Source
p.50 Marilyn Angel Wynn/Nativestock Pictures
p.51 (l) George Rodger/Magnum; (r) David Davies/Press Association Images
p.69 Erich Auerbach/Getty Images
p.73 Corbis
p.78 Ronald Wittek/Picture Press
p.85 The Society of Teachers of the Alexander Technique, London